Waiting for Cancer to Come

Waiting for Cancer to Come

Women's Experiences with
Genetic Testing and Medical Decision Making
for Breast and Ovarian Cancer

Sharlene Hesse-Biber

The University of Michigan Press
Ann Arbor

Published in the United States of America by
The University of Michigan Press
Manufactured in the United States of America
⊗ Printed on acid-free paper

2017   2016   2015   2014   4   3   2   1

A CIP catalog record for this book is available from the British Library.

Library of Congress Cataloging-in-Publication Data

Hesse-Biber, Sharlene Nagy

Waiting for cancer to come : women's experiences with genetic testing & medical decision making for breast and ovarian cancer / Sharlene Hesse-Biber.
      p.   cm.
   Includes bibliographical references and index.
   ISBN 978-0-472-07219-4 (hardcover : alk. paper)—ISBN 978-0-472-05219-6 (pbk. : alk. paper)—ISBN 978-0-472-12035-2 (e-book)
   I. Title.
   [DNLM: 1. Genetic Testing—Personal Narratives.   2. Hereditary Breast and Ovarian Cancer Syndrome—genetics—Personal Narratives.
3. Decision Making—Personal Narratives.   4. Women's Health—Personal Narratives. WP 870]
   RC280.B8   2014
   616.99'449042—dc23
                                                    2014005568

To my incredible and courageous sister,
JANET GREEN FISCHER,
with love and remembrance.

Contents

Acknowledgments

First, my thanks go to the inspirational women who participated in the interviews for my study, who bravely agreed to share their experiences of genetic testing and the myriad of medical decision making they confronted on their BRCA journey. Their courage, wisdom, and willingness to share their stories with me—and my readers—is tremendously appreciated. I am extremely honored by their presence in this research project.

Many thanks to the Boston College community that contributed generously to this project. I want to especially thank Dr. David Karp, Professor of Sociology, Boston College, for his expert advice throughout the various stages of this research project. I also want to extend my gratitude to Boston College's Office of Research Administration for providing research grants to support this project. In particular, I wish to thank Dean William Petri for his support and encouragement as I continued forward on my research journey.

I am grateful to Karen Taylor's careful reading of the manuscript and her insightful editorial suggestions. Special thanks also go to Boston College undergraduates, Alicia Johnson, class of 2010; Elizabeth Jekanowski, class of 2013; and Mary Downer, class of 2011. They each brought unique intuition and inspiration to the project. Their excellent research skills and editorial assistance with chapter revisions and data analysis provided me with insights and consensual validation of my research findings.

Along the way, many others supported and assisted in this project and I am particularly grateful to the enthusiastic support and dedicated efforts of Boston College undergraduate Hilary Flowers, class of 2009; and Jennifer Hotaling, graduate student in the School of Education at Boston College, class of 2013.

I am grateful to my daughters, Sarah Alexandra and Julia Ariel, for their patience, humor, love, kindness, and enthusiastic support for my combining my work and family lives. Thanks also go to my mother, Helene Stockert; my sister, Georgia Gerraghty; and my brother, Charles Nagy.

I want to express my sincere appreciation to my husband, Michael Peter Biber, MD, for "hanging in there" while I spent many hours on this project. His support, love, and understanding were crucial during all phases of this writing project.

Sharlene Hesse-Biber

Prologue

Sitting with BRCA is like being a character in Samuel Beckett's play
  Waiting for Godot,
Being in a place where time becomes waiting.
Waiting for cancer to come.
"Not if I get cancer, but when I get cancer."
Wanting to act, yet feeling immobilized, unable to move forward.
Feeling like "my breasts are ticking time bombs."
Waiting for cancer to come.

Plotting and pleading with cancer.
"Playing Russian roulette with my cancer."
"Asking God to deal with it,
He will tell me what to do."
"Following my mother's cancer clock."
I can hear my mother saying, "Don't wait to get cancer."
Waiting for cancer to come.

I'm going to "Kill it." "Stab it." "Cut it out." "Talk to it."
"I'm going to bargain with it."
I "brushed it off."
I'm trying to get to a place where I don't feel under siege.
I'm trying very hard to outwit the BRCA mutation gene.
"I really wanted to take control."
Waiting for cancer to come.

What to do? What else?
I'm "screwed no matter what."

Denying it.
Living with it.
Watching it.
Keeping it under control.
"Impending doom"—"I guess I die."
Waiting for cancer to come.

Playing the statistical odds of my cancer risk.
My odds of getting cancer are my magical numbers.
"Fact-finding."
Becoming a trailblazer and creating my path to treatment.
"I thought I would never do that, are they crazy?"
No one to guide me.
I join together with my online BRCA sisterhood.
Waiting for cancer to come.

When to get tested? "I don't want to know, but I know."
"I don't want to know, but I plan my life around cancer, but I don't
    want to know about it."
"Every day is full of pain and terror."
"I decide when to know."
"I already know it, but don't want to know it."
"How could I not end up with cancer?"
Waiting for cancer to come.

Being in a luminal space that helps me to feel empowered.
One that allows me to still feel like a woman.
"I want to date. I want a boyfriend."
"Will he feel my breasts and discover they are hard and cold?"
"When to tell him I have the BRCA gene?"
"I want to get married and have a family."
Waiting for cancer to come.

"I couldn't get my surgery scheduled fast enough."
"If I want a boyfriend, a husband, a family, I've got to look normal."
"I want to be a woman." "Maybe nipple sparing will make me look
    more normal."
Instead of normal, at least, "I'll get a bonus from my mastectomy"
"I can get bigger breasts."

"I can have my surgeon do a tummy tuck."
"Maybe my surgeon can take the fat from my stomach and stuff it
    into my breasts."
"This is what I want to do."
"I want them to look more normal." "I wanted them to look natural."
Waiting for cancer to come.

"My husband won't look at my breasts. He doesn't touch me the way
    he used to after surgery."
"I want to go back to normal, the way things were. It's my new
    normal."
"BRCA doesn't mean that much to me anymore. BRCA is what
    happened, and it will fade from my life."
"I'm cancer free."
"I still look like me."
"I'm fine." "Nothing's wrong."
"Everything is fine."
"I feel whole, I feel well."
"I had BRCA, but now I don't."
"I feel normal again."
"It won't be back."
"I have time"
Waiting for cancer to come.

What to do with a positive diagnosis?
Who to tell? When to tell?
Needing to keep BRCA a secret from family members, friends.
Not being connected to family makes it difficult to talk about the bad
    news.
"Most people don't want to talk with you about it, my sister, and
    mother for instance."
"I became an outcast in my family."

"Nobody understands why I'm doing this—taking off healthy
    breasts."
"Everything I did, I was thinking about my daughter."
"I'd rather have BRCA than a family member, especially my sister."
"Maybe we all have it?"
"It's all in our family."

"It's spreading across the generations. Me, my sister, my mother and
   grandmother."
"Maybe my children have it."
"I would never want my family to go through all this."
"By the time my children are grown, they will find a cure, I'm sure."
Are we all waiting for cancer to come?

"My ovaries? Well that's for forty."
"I have ten more years to wait. I'm waiting for it. The day for them to
   come out."
"My doctor says by forty you won't have 'em."
"Yeah, they're going to come out, but now, I have some time."
"No, knowing all this doesn't interfere with my time line."
"My husband? He says maybe we should have more kids now. Have
   our family then get my ovaries out after that. Maybe. . . ."
"I have time."
"That's the BRCA way!" BRCA? What's that?
Still waiting for cancer to come.

This poetic reflection comes from the voices of women who have shared
with me their emotions, challenges, and hopes since learning that they are
carriers of a devastating genetic mutation—BRCA. This mutation places
them at high risk for developing breast, ovarian, and other cancers. So
BRCA-positive women are in a state of waiting. They wait because they are
not ready to take the genetic test. They wait to hear test results. They mustn't
wait too long before having preventative surgery. Mostly, they wait for the
next breakthrough that will free their children from cancer's grip.

Some women tell me they already knew they had the mutation but didn't
want to be tested until they were ready to know. For some women, cancer
has already struck. It threatens them or someone within their own families.
It's taken the lives of loved ones—a mother, a sister, a father, a brother. For
some, cancer's path crosses the generations, going back in time to claim
the lives of grandmothers, grandfathers, aunts, cousins, and second cousins. These family histories and the BRCA-positive mutation status of family
members often make women aware of their cancer risk and lead them to be
tested. Being tested for a genetic mutation is an affirmation and relief for
some women, letting them finally know what they already knew—they are
BRCA positive.

Other women come to a positive test result by chance, never expecting that they are carriers of the BRCA mutation. They have little or no family history of cancer and are the first within their families to make known what may have been unknown for generations. Some have no access to the cancer history of their families, having had past generations murdered during the Nazi regime.

The cacophony of women's voices that swirl around one another in the opening poem captures the genetic testing experience and the myriad ways women come to terms with their genetic news. Women with the BRCA mutation have feelings that collide, affirm, and connect; they express anger, sadness, and resignation. Some women repeat the voice of authority, accepting what their doctors tell them to feel and do. Others voice the concerns of loved ones: husbands, mothers, sisters, best friends, and life partners. And still others forge their own paths, making bold and difficult decisions despite or in conjunction with advice.

I came to realize, too, that this poem touches on the many stages of the various BRCA experiences that women go through and continue to pass through in seeking a space where they feel healed and empowered to move forward with their lives. I hear the voices of grief over the death of loved ones, over the physical loss of breasts and ovaries. I hear despair and isolation. I hear fighting words, too. Some women are warriors who wage battle against their inherited cancer risk. Others bargain with their cancer diagnosis or fate or God as a way to buy some time. Some women seek ways to feel "cancer free" and immediately launch into surgery in order to escape the fear of getting cancer. Others express the hope of moving toward a "new normal," a place where they feel whole again and where they create a life that is not held hostage by their genetic mutation.

This book takes you on a journey through the life experiences of these women. It provides a critical analytic window on the impact of genetic testing on women and their families. I spoke with women who tested positive for the BRCA1 or BRCA2 mutation, which increases an individual's risk for breast, ovarian, and other cancers, such as pancreatic cancer. This occurs because the BRCA1 gene is located on chromosome 17, and BRCA2 is on chromosome 13. These particular genes function to abate the onset of cancer, so when they mutate, women are at higher risk of developing breast and/ or ovarian cancer. The test for these inherited genetic mutations has been available since the early 1990s. Women with BRCA mutations (BRCA is an acronym for BReast CAncer) have a lifetime risk (based on a life expectancy of 85 years) of developing breast cancer that ranges from 60 to 90 percent for BRCA1 and 30 to 85 percent for BRCA2. These lifetime risk assessments are dramatically lower (at 12 percent) for women who do not carry this genetic mutation marker.

Women now have access to biotechnological tools derived from the Human Genome Project and fueled by a genetic-testing industry that promises the consumer a crystal ball able to illumine the potential diseases lying dormant within their bodies. Such genetic tests are framed by the testing industry as vital preventive knowledge, as tools by which women, in particular, can preempt genetic disorders before they strike. These new technologies have fueled an increasingly "at-risk" society as they intervene in our lives to reveal more medical risks and perpetuate the growth in "expert knowledge" and other new technologies necessary to manage this risk (Beck 1992; Giddens 1990; Lupton 1999). While the BRCA test is prohibitively expensive for many women, the market for such testing continues to grow, as consumers with the means to employ genetic testing for particular mutations see it a means to address future medical risks. All kinds of genetic tests are under development, and genetic testing kits are becoming more readily available over the Internet and without a prescription from a doctor. Genetic testing is rapidly becoming a routine part of staying healthy by preventing disease. At least, that is how genetic testing websites frame these tests. Why wouldn't you want to know what genetic disorders you might be at risk for? While at it, why not test everyone in your family? In fact, the testing industry is beginning to market genetic tests to a younger and younger population.

If we think of the testing industry as just that, an industry, we can begin to see a collusion of economic interests. Not only testing companies but also other enterprises benefit economically from positive testing results, as many costly medical tests and procedures often follow each positive diagnosis. Still, isn't more health information better?

As our journey through the lives of women who have already been genetically tested will show, it's not that simple. Between 2009 and 2011, I interviewed sixty-four women who tested positive for the BRCA mutation. I wanted to explore their lived experiences with genetic testing and all the consequences of a positive result. Their stories are the foundation of this book, and its quotations are their voices, taken directly from the interviews. You will also find demographic statistics about the women I spoke with. These are the results of an online survey sent to each woman I interviewed. A more elaborate research description and explanation of this study is contained in the epilogue.

Once they open up the genetic testing Pandora's box, women and their families begin to find their lives altered in complex ways: emotionally, socially, economically, and psychologically. The following account encapsulates, in many ways, the dilemmas, hopes, and concerns of women who undergo genetic testing for the BRCA mutation. But all stories are both emblematic and exceptional.

A Vial of Blood: A Dying Sister's Legacy

Jessica (all names are pseudonyms, and I have slightly changed a number of identifying details to protect confidentiality) knew something was not right about her younger sister Mary's sudden onset of inflammatory breast cancer. And she was right. Mary died at the age of thirty-seven, just fifteen months after her cancer diagnosis.

Just prior to her diagnosis, Mary was widowed. Her husband had died suddenly of heart disease. Jessica recalls other troubling events happening around the time her sister became ill. Mary was just laid off from her job and was living in Colorado with her two young children. Things really went downhill when Mary felt something "terribly wrong" with her breast, but, because of the expensive insurance payments, she had given up her health insurance shortly after she lost her sales job. As Jessica recalls, "My sister waited for things to turn around in her life, but they didn't, and so she was in a bit of a state of denial about what was going on with her breast situation." She visited a doctor several months later and found out she had a very aggressive type of breast cancer that needed to be treated immediately.

Having little money for adequate treatment, Mary decided to move to Florida to live with her sister. Jessica and her husband took care of Mary's children and also agreed to help Mary navigate the medical system in their state in order to find the cancer treatment she needed.

At that time, Jessica and Mary never made any connection between Mary's cancer and the possibility of Mary being BRCA positive. After all, no one they knew had been diagnosed with or died from breast or ovarian cancer, although there was some history of other cancers on both sides of their family. It was not until Jessica's sister developed an aggressive form of inflammatory breast cancer that Jessica began to be concerned. Why? Where had it come from? Yet no medical personnel alerted either of them that they might need to be tested for hereditary breast cancer.

Mary died in the hospital while undergoing treatment for her illness. Right before her sister's death, Jessica decided to look up more information about Mary's specific type of breast cancer. She used a computer in the hospital waiting area, a short distance from Mary's room. What Jessica discovered on the Internet was that early age onset of breast cancer might signal a hereditary condition. Upon learning of Mary's death minutes later, Jessica wondered whether or not her sister's blood or tissue should be sampled and tested for the BRCA mutation. Yet there were no medical staff members who thought she should do so when she queried them. They claimed, instead, that a "range of crazy coincidences" caused Mary's sudden onset of inflammatory breast cancer. But, luckily, Jessica found a more receptive doctor.

> Just by coincidence, there was a resident in the room where we were using the computer and he said, "You know, that's my department, let me see what I can find." And he found that someone had taken a vial of her blood that morning. So he put in me in touch with the genetics department, and they expedited getting that blood processed for testing.

A sister's legacy to her family was that vial of blood. It was sent out to the Myriad Corporation, a genetic testing company located in Utah. Jessica paid $3,300 dollars of her own money to test her sister's blood, which came back positive for the BRCA mutation. Jessica was then tested and was also positive. Within six months, in her early forties, Jessica had her ovaries and uterus removed, and, about four months later, she had a bilateral breast removal.

Witnessing a family member experience breast cancer, especially if it is fatal, can be a strong factor pushing women to have breast or ovarian surgery as a preventive strategy, rather than pursuing surveillance of those organs most susceptible to cancer. As Jessica notes, "I didn't see the point in waiting to be a cancer patient. It was insane for me not to take advantage of the heads-up that I had. I also wanted to show my daughters that it's not the end of the world—you can do something about it and make it through."

Jessica is now a role model and advisor for the rest of her family. Many BRCA patients become examples and advisors, showing the rest of their families how to deal with a BRCA mutation. As Jessica notes, "I'm the oldest of the siblings. I have become the one that everybody kind of comes to. I keep everybody informed and up to date." Jessica feels a moral obligation to fill this advisory role, explaining that she performs it "in the memory of my sister." She is especially worried about her younger brother having a genetic mutation. He refuses to be tested. "It's a weakness to succumb to medical procedures," he thinks. Jessica hopes her brother will eventually change his mind and agree to be tested in order to protect his own children.

She expresses her emotions the most when talking about how being BRCA positive will affect her children's, as well as her nieces' and nephews' generation. She has already told her brother's teenage daughter that her father has a 50 percent chance of testing positive. Jessica's oldest child, who is about to turn fifteen, has also been informed about her family's history with BRCA and the importance of getting tested down the road. It is critical to protect the next generation by informing young people early, Jessica believes, even if it takes time for them to fully comprehend the implications of a BRCA-positive diagnosis. She acknowledges that perhaps her brother thinks she is overstepping her role by telling the next generation of family members more than their own parents wanted them to know; however, she justifies informing her young relatives by saying she is "not going to lie to them" for the sake of their parents not wanting to tell the truth.

Jessica is taking on the role of BRCA informer, carrying out what she feels is a critical mission to serve her family. She uses militaristic terminology to describe her experiences and aims, noting that, although her sister "didn't know what hit and struck her and gave her cancer," she, Jessica, is now "armed with information." She imagines herself battling the bad cancer genes. She won't be "ambushed" by them, as her sister was.

Her battle hasn't always been easy. Several breast-reconstruction surgeries have left her deeply dissatisfied with her breasts. Her first breast surgeon told her he wanted to try a new type of implant called "gummy bear implants." These contain a form of cohesive gel, which caused postoperative infections and severe breast pain. Both are still with Jessica today. After explaining these side effects to her surgeon, she discovered that medical staff members call her "the headache patient." She never did get an adequate response from her surgeon.

This negative experience got her thinking. She decided that the surgeons who cared for her were almost in a "brotherhood" and often placed their loyalty to one another above commitment to their patients. Jessica switched her surgery clinic and notes how much more doctors and staff listen to her concerns. They reconstructed her breasts to her satisfaction, telling her they would not stop until "it's right with her." She is currently very happy with her breast reconstruction, and she has a high degree of trust in her new surgeons, trust they have earned.

Jessica has experienced firsthand the power of her bad genes and continues to survey her body closely for any signs of BRCA-related disease. Recently, her surgeon removed a tumor from her knee and polyps from her colon. She is now under surveillance for these conditions as well. As she explains, she can't help but feel sometimes that her bad genes will always continue to wage war on her body. Her BRCA-testing experience led Jessica to examine the history of cancer and other diseases in her family tree more fully, and she actually discovered that several family members had died at young ages from heart failure on her father's side of the family.

Keeping watch over her family's bad genes has become an all-encompassing task for Jessica, a task that includes watching over her own body, hoping that her bad genes will not claim yet another one of her organs.

Jessica's story is particularly poignant for me. I also lost my younger sister, Janet, to an aggressive form of breast cancer. It wasn't until several years later that I, too, developed breast cancer, as did my older sister, who was diagnosed with the disease a year later. It was as if breast cancer was raining down hard on my siblings. How could this happen? I did not know of a strong history of breast or ovarian cancer in my family. My oncologist suggested that my older sister and I get tested for the BRCA 1 and BRCA 2 genetic mutations. It was then that reality set in: Could I have a genetic mutation? What did that mean, and how could I wrap my mind around how this news would affect my two daughters?

It was with great trepidation that my sister and I decided to get tested together at the Dana-Farber Cancer Institute in Boston, Massachusetts. On the designated day, we enter the clinic together and wait for our blood to be drawn. Most of the women around us appear to be at various stages in their breast or ovarian cancer treatment. Some were already showing signs of the ravages of chemotherapy. They wear brightly colored bandanas to cover their hair loss. The wrists of others sprouted IV ports held in place with brightly colored strips of medical tape, signifying that they are waiting to enter the infusion room for yet another seven hours or so of chemotherapy treatment.

Waiting to get tested, I recall being in this very room several years ago with my younger sister, who had flown up from Virginia to obtain a second opinion about how to best treat her aggressive breast cancer. I remember how much time I, too, have already spent on my own cancer treatment. I'd just finished a course of five-days-a-week radiation treatments in the sub-basement of this same building.

Waiting in this room again makes me think that, if any one of us should test positive, it should be me and not my older sister. When my older sister was diagnosed with breast cancer, she reacted with total terror. Having cancer felt like a death sentence. She was sure she was going to die. Having a younger sister die from breast cancer had already taken a toll on our family, and I think that, once my older sister was diagnosed, she used our younger sister's cancer history narrative to guide her own sense of how things would go.

We give our blood, leave, and wait some more. Three weeks later we get our test results back, and I visit a genetics counselor, who seems to be reading from some type of script: "The DNA analysis did not reveal a detectable BRCA1 or BRCA2 gene alteration." Leaving the genetics office, I feel I've dodged the bad cancer gene. Several days later, I get an official letter from The Dana-Farber Cancer Institute summarizing my counseling session. I'm struck by the official interpretation of the negative result, an interpretation that sends chills and fear throughout my body. The good news of this letter—there is no detectable gene alteration. However, unbeknownst to me even after my conversation with the genetics counselor, there are three possible ways to interpret a negative result. First, my cancer could be related to a "combination of genetic and environment factors."

The second interpretation, described as "unlikely," is that I have "an alteration in BRCA1 or BRCA2, but the laboratory was unable to find it based on the types of analysis that were performed." I stop reading the letter at this point, not knowing how to understand this second explanation. I ask myself, "Didn't I just get tested for BRCA1 and 2?" The answer is yes, and no. As the letter goes on to say, "The laboratory has recently added another component to their testing to try and detect large changes in BRCA1 and BRCA2 that would not have been found with the testing that was performed on you." Apparently, the probability of this being the case in families with a strong history of breast cancer is between 1 and 3 percent. If I want to put my mind at ease, however, I will need to pay $650 out of pocket for this new test. My insurance company is unlikely to pay the additional expense. What is my immediate reaction? This second option, I think, is a clever scam so the genetic testing industry can make more money by provoking uncertainty, even among those who receive a "negative" result! The third interpretation of my negative result is also frightening. My breast cancer could have been caused by an alteration in a *different* cancer susceptibility gene.

So, what to make of the letter? I want to cling to the good news, but, as I reread the letter, I begin to feel some doubt and concern about what it means to have a negative result. The reality of the matter is stark. We three sisters have all received the breast cancer diagnosis, and, given my strong family history of other cancers, I could still be carrying a genetic mutation.

I'm terrified to tell my older sister about this possibility because she also received a negative result and was told by her genetics counselor in New York that she has little to worry about. Upon hearing this good news, my sister expressed an outpouring of relief. So why should I rain down yet more uncertainty on her? Why bring the possibility that she may still be at risk of having a genetic mutation into the picture right now?

A year after being tested, I find out that scientists are continuing to isolate two other genes, BRCA3 and BRCA4, which may also be linked to hereditary breast cancers. Should both of us get tested for these genes down the road?

Looking back on my testing experience, I feel a bit cheated, overall. Why can't I get a definitive negative result? Why must I live with the small risk that I could be a BRCA carrier? I ask myself whether I will get tested again once other tests become available. But how much testing is really going to tell me finally and definitively that I have no hereditary risk? Is there yet another "bad" gene in the future that I'll have to worry about? Besides, being at risk for a genetic mutation is an issue not only for me but also for those I am bound to by blood—those within my family tree. Do I need to tell all my family members to get tested just to be on the safe side?

One thing has become clear to me, as it has for many of the women I've interviewed while writing this book: life is never the same once you open up the genetic testing box. Even if your curiosity is rewarded by the good news of a negative result, opening up the possibility of inheriting cancer begins to transform lives.

As the women of this book tell their stories, we see how disruptive genetic testing can be. Test results can rip open a family and lay bare many difficult family dilemmas. Genetic testing may serve to separate emotionally those in the family who have the gene from those who do not. Some family members choose to keep their positive status a secret and suffer in silence, ashamed to bring such bad news to their loved ones. Other "bad-gene" carriers feel a moral obligation to tell all their relatives. But, as was the case for Jessica, family members on the receiving end can see this information as unwelcome news and the person who delivers it as interfering, or worse. Some family members just don't want to know, and permanent rifts can occur as a result of testing revelations.

This book focuses on the lived experiences of women who have tested positive for the BRCA gene and on how their lives have evolved in response to a positive diagnosis. We examine the diverse medical decision pathways they take, before, during, and after testing, and we consider how they, as single, married, or divorced women with or without children, respond to the challenge of being a BRCA-mutation carrier. We look at how a positive diagnosis upends some lives, creating in women a sense of disempowerment and despair, but also at how others come to terms with a positive result and create a new sense of empowerment and positive change within their individual and family lives.

We delve into family dynamics involved when a daughter, mother, sister, wife, or extended family member receives a positive test result. We discuss the keeping of secrets and what impact telling or not telling has on the unity of families within and across generations. We also look at what being BRCA positive means to this diverse group of women. In what ways does a positive result affect a woman's sense of self? Does a positive result lead to the surgical removal of breasts, ovaries, or both? When does that occur?

We also take a step back to look at the genetic testing industry and at its role in these women's lives. The experiences of the women who spoke with me are embedded in a multibillion-dollar testing and surgical culture in which a number of powerful interest groups have a stake. The genetic testing industry and the medical profession have constructed a new preventive frame around getting tested not only for the BRCA mutation but also for an array of genetic factors correlated with medical conditions. The push for preventive measures supports a culture of fear in regards to the potential for future medical issues. As demonstrated in this book, this fear leads many women to equate their BRCA-positive mutation status with a cancer diagnosis. Jessica, for example, feels that knowing her BRCA status has freed her from what she interprets as her genetic destiny. Increasingly, surgery is becoming seen as the only pathway to eradicate cancer risk.

This book provides the reader with a window onto the growing impact and normalization of genetic testing in the United States. It also has things to say about the biomedical surveillance of women's bodies and the commercialization of health care. In America, consumers are rapidly taking up the "prevention and choice" rhetoric surrounding testing and are demanding access to testing for a range of genetic mutations, from which they hope to save themselves by purchasing various other medical services. We also look at the emergence of one's genetic status as a new somatic or body-based identity and see how the testing experience can be both empowering and disempowering for women.

We end our journey by pulling together the strands of wisdom gathered from listening closely to the experiences of women who have crossed over the testing line. What are the policy implications of knowing about these women's lived experiences? How should we make use of their insights regarding the organization of the genetic testing industry as a whole, the ways in which counselors and medical professionals deliver genetic information, and the current treatment protocols for BRCA-positive women? The women I interviewed provide us with concrete and various paths to change. But these paths all head in one direction—the medical and testing industries need to create systems and information that better serve to empower women as they assess their genetic risk and navigate treatment options in order to reduce their risk of developing cancer.

ONE

The Genetic Testing Industry

Capitalizing on Fear, Selling Empowerment

One day, Heather is riding home from work on the subway when she notices an advertisement: "Are you ready to fight disease before it starts?" The ad encourages her to learn more about the BRAC*Analysis*® test for the BRCA1/2 gene mutations that indicate a woman's increased risk of developing breast and ovarian cancer. Heather is twenty-two years old and has a family history of breast cancer. The ad strikes a nerve and raises new questions. Can this test really help her fight disease? Should Heather consider it? Will it let her know, once and for all, what her risk is of getting breast cancer—and how to deal with it?

Many of us have seen advertising like this in subways, magazines, and online. Not only for the BRCA test but many other genetic tests. The genetic testing industry has grown into a multibillion-dollar business. Profits depend an ever-expanding base of women and men seeking the test. Online genetic testing companies have also surged recently. Their claims are often overstated and they lack any governmental or medical oversight on the quality of the tests or the legitimacy of these companies' claims (Hogarth, Javitt, and Melzer 2008; Shuren 2010). In fact, according to the U.S. Food and Drug Administration (FDA), many companies haven't established a firm causal link between someone's test results and her actual risk of developing disease. No genetic tests offered directly to consumers (that is, not through a doctor, but directly from a company) have been reviewed by the FDA to determine whether they are medically reliable, accurate, or meaningful to the patient. So why are so many women getting tested?

The sheer number of genetic tests available is growing dramatically. Tests for more than 1,200 diseases are currently available clinically, and hundreds more are offered in research settings (Hogarth, Javitt, and Melzer 2008). Genetic testing is becoming more and more normal procedure among medical professionals and individual consumers. The trend is fueled by the growing commercialization of the testing industry and its potential for increased profits. Tests are even moving out of specialized clinicians' offices and are marketed directly to general practitioners and their patients (McCabe and McCabe 2004). Today, the genetic testing industry is worth billions of dollars. In 2007, one of its leading companies, Myriad Genetics, earned $145.3 million in revenue from its molecular diagnostic tests alone (Liu and Pearson 2008; Thrush and McCaffrey 2010).

The high cost of each test keeps business booming. For example, up until recently, the Myriad Corporation had cornered the BRCA genetic testing market (until the Supreme Court struck down its monopoly on BRCA testing in June 2013 claiming that human genes cannot be patented) and was charging between three and five thousand dollars to test for the BRCA1/2 gene mutations. This is a cost women must bear—women and their families. Many health insurance companies are reluctant to pay for this sort of genetic testing, especially because a positive test result could lead to the even greater costs of preventive surveillance or surgeries. No wonder, then, that an extraordinary amount of money is moving straight from consumers to genetic testing companies, which have been expanding as rapidly as technological developments allow. The genetic testing industry is growing thanks to millions of women who are waiting for cancer to come and willing to pay for the test.

But the BRCA test is only a small part of the industry's direct-to-customer offerings. Now anyone can get tested for a wide variety of potentially harmful gene mutations. They can even arrange for an entire scan of their genomes (Burke 2004; Thrush and Ruth 2010). In fact, the growth of the genetic testing industry has outpaced the ability of FDA regulators to oversee the quality of genetic tests and the company's advertisements (Geransar and Einsiedal 2008; Shuren 2010). Since the FDA began to monitor these companies in 2003, the increasing number of genetic tests available has made it even more difficult for the FDA to regulate them (Companies and Markets 2011).

The excessive and fear-based marketing these companies use is another concern of the FDA. Although those with potentially life-threatening gene mutations may benefit from hearing about these tests, some may feel undue pressure to be tested and to have their children tested as well (Liu and Pearson 2008). Several genetic testing companies use this sense of familial duty and exploit in their marketing campaigns the moral obligation parents feel toward their children.

Who benefits from genetic testing? Does concern for profits blind corporations to the ways these tests affect the lives of those who purchase and use them? To what extent do individuals understand the range of social, economic, and psychological implications of getting a genetic test? We explore these questions by considering the experiences of women who have undergone genetic testing for the BRCA mutations for breast and ovarian cancer, by looking at their perceptions of what it means to undergo genetic testing and their expectations of how it will affect them and their families. To what extent do these perceptions and expectations about genetic testing mirror the marketing messages of the genetic testing industry?

The Coming of Age of Genetic Testing

To start, let's take a quick look at the history of the ever-growing genetic testing industry. The purpose of this book is to share women's voices and women's stories—but their voices must be heard in the context of the medical and commercial world of genetic testing. No person's voice is not in some way shaped by the people and institutions around them. And this is certainly true in the world of BRCA testing.

The well-educated woman living in the United States in 1990 would probably have known that each person's DNA contains a complex and unique genetic blueprint. She might even have understood that predispositions to particular illnesses, as well as other things such as eye and hair color, can be passed on from parents to children through inherited genetic material. But genetic testing was in its infancy then. After all, the first person in the United States ever convicted as a result of DNA evidence was sentenced in 1987. But our knowledge of genes and of genetic testing was going to expand quickly in the last decade before the millennium, in part as a consequence of the Human Genome Project. This international effort began in 1990 to map and understand the function of each human gene and its location on a given chromosome. By 2003, the project was complete. Knowing this information about human genetics was a critical step in the development of genetic testing.

As the Human Genome Project mapped more of our genetic structure, researchers discovered specific gene mutations, especially those that could be passed on from parent to child. Concerned parents and society were looking to new technologies for ways to screen for inherited diseases that would later need to be managed. Over the past decade, the genetic testing of aspiring parents and prenatal testing have become increasingly widespread, especially for conditions such as Down syndrome.

In the 1980s, Mary-Claire King and her colleagues identified a gene mutation in the region of chromosome 17, later known as BRCA1, that placed women at high risk for developing breast and especially ovarian cancer. A 1990 report of this genetic discovery known as "breast cancer gene," set the stage for a rapid commercial development of a genetic testing for BRCA1. Myriad Genetics, a biopharmaceutical and genomics company founded in 1991, moved quickly to develop a genetic test for BRCA1, and subsequently mapping a genetic segment on chromosome 13 known as BRCA2, found to also predispose women to higher breast and ovarian cancer risk. It discovered the genes tied to breast and ovarian cancer by linking genealogical information it gathered from Mormon families in Utah to the medical records from Utah cancer registries. Myriad obtained the sole patent rights to these genes and began to offer the BRAC*Analysis* test commercially. The test diagnoses inherited susceptibility for breast and ovarian cancer and is now available in countries around the world. By obtaining, in 1998, patents to control both the research and commercial uses of the BRCA1 gene, Myriad cornered the market and prevented any competitors from performing the test. It soon gained similar patent rights over the BRCA2 gene (Gold and Carbone 2010). Yet, up until the recent Supreme Court ruling in June 2013 that struck down Myriad's patent claims, Myriad had subjected its competitors to high-cost litigation for violating its exclusive patent rights to these specific gene mutations.

In 1996, Myriad began to market its test as a $900 kit sold directly to consumers. However, the testing kit was quickly taken off the market as a result of severe criticism from the medical community. Many health-care professionals argued that selling such a test directly to the consumer was harmful. Trained genetic counselors or other knowledgeable experts should deliver the test results, they claimed. Myriad reissued the BRAC*Analysis* test with a new requirement: consumers must convince their health-care providers to act as intermediaries by ordering the test and providing genetic counseling (Williams-Jones 2006). This still stands—women must get the test from a medical professional, and not directly from Myriad. The cost of a BRAC-*Analysis* test can vary depending on how much detail a consumer wants. Current rates for comprehensive genetic tests are around $2,600, with an additional $1,100 for a rapid test return. The company offers slightly reduced rates to family members who wish to be tested.

Health-care groups and consumer advocates often argue that Myriad's monopoly on BRCA testing has made these tests overly expensive. Many oppose the patenting of human genes in general and, more specifically, the patenting of genes used in diagnostic tests. These patents may keep other researchers from discovering new information. Many researchers think that scientists have avoided publicizing their discoveries because they fear infringing upon Myriad's patents (Gold and Carbone 2010). They can make genetic tests more expensive, which can potentially increase the cost of health care (Gold and Carbone 2010). And as I mentioned before, insurers are often unwilling to cover the high cost of these tests, which may stop many people from being tested (Klitzman 2010).

With these issues in mind, the American Civil Liberties Union (ACLU) and the Public Patent Foundation (PUBPAT) filed a lawsuit against Myriad in May 2009. (International opposition, including challenges to Myriad's European patents, occurred much earlier and has since had ripple effects on American legislation.) The ACLU charged that patents related to breast and ovarian cancers are unconstitutional and prohibit further research into life-saving medicine and women's treatment options (American Civil Liberties Union 2012). In March of the following year, the New York District Court held that "a product of nature," such as a gene, cannot be patented, deeming a portion of Myriad's seven patents invalid (Trusso 2010). Myriad filed a notice of appeal in June 2010 in the U.S. Court of Appeals for the Federal Circuit, and, in July 2011, the appeals court ruled in favor of Myriad's patent, saying that the genes are different enough when isolated from the body to not to be considered a product of nature. The closely watched case finally reached the Supreme Court in March 2012, when an appeals court was ordered to reconsider its decision to uphold the patents in response to a recent ruling on a similar blood test that could not be patented (Pollack 2012). Meanwhile in 2012, the ACLU launched an online campaign called Take Back Our Genes that raised awareness about the case and encourages women to share their stories (Gay 2012).

In June 2013, the U.S. Supreme Court ruled against Myriad corporation's BRCA gene patent claim by voting unanimously that no company can patent an isolated human gene. However, the Supreme Court also ruled that a company can patent a synthetically created genetic substance called cDNA. The good news is that Myriad Corporation may now face some stiff competition in the marketplace that will drive down the current price of a BRCA genetic test. However, in order to protect its competitive advantage, in a press release dated September 5, 2013, the Myriad Corporation announced the graduated role of its new "multi-gene" genetic test called myRisk™. This new product includes testing for twenty-five genes associated with eight hereditary cancers that encompass testing for genetic mutations for breast, colorectal, ovarian, endometrial, pancreatic, prostate, gastric, and melanoma. Myriad is said to see this new test as a replacement for its primary revenue generating BRAC*Analysis* test. The price for the myRisk test ranges from $4,000–$4,500. The myRisk test may not be subjected to the Supreme Court's gene patent ruling. Myriad continues to retain its right to withhold important genetic test results stored in their large privately owned genetic database used by Myriad to "norm" and thereby interpret the meaning of individual genetic test results. It remains to be seen if and when Myriad's competitors get access to this comparative genetic information.

Even given these new initiatives by Myriad Corporation to maintain its market share and competitive advantage since the U.S. Supreme Court's decision, one important outcome for women who test positive for the BRCA1 and BRCA2 mutation is that there is a way for them to verify their test results by getting a second opinion before they decide to undergo preventative surgeries. Given the opening up of the genetic testing marketplace, women and especially women of color may now be offered testing for a range of genes also found to be associated with hereditary breast and ovarian cancer, beyond BRCA1 and BRCA2, allowing a more complete understanding of BRCA1 and 2 mutation carrier's overall hereditary cancer risk.

Bringing the Test to You

While the legal battle in the Supreme Court has decided against the patenting of genes, up until this time and still ongoing, Myriad has taken advantage and continues to push its unique position in the industry to further market the BRAC*Analysis* test as well as its upcoming new BRCA test that does not appear to be subjected to the Supreme Court 2013 patent ruling. In the 1990s, Myriad promoted its tests successfully to physicians and patients through the company's website and direct outreach. The company entered into what are essentially sales agreements with major insurance companies and health care providers, giving them comprehensive educational—that is, marketing—materials (Gold and Carbone 2010; Pollack 2007; Williams-Jones 2006). Beginning in 2007, Myriad Genetics turned this outreach into a direct-to-consumer (DTC) advertising campaign, bringing information about the BRCA1/2 test directly to the public. The campaign was launched in the northeastern United States with television ads. It framed BRAC*Analysis* as the route to preventing disease and the way to take control of one's health. Myriad's president at the time, Gregory Critchfield, commented on the campaign: "The purpose of the BRAC*Analysis* public awareness campaign is to save lives. The risks of breast and ovarian cancers are very high in individuals carrying mutations in either the BRCA1 or BRCA2 genes." He continued by claiming that high-risk women would benefit from this testing because they could now "take steps to reduce their risk for these cancers" (Myriad Genetics 2007b).

Many women agree. The BRCA test is a means of gaining the knowledge a woman needs to take action against cancer. For these women, knowledge is power. And the knowledge of their gene mutation lets them make choices about how to manage their health. Carrie knew she was at risk for cancer but sick of waiting for cancer to come. She said, "Why have this hang over my head all the time? And so, I said, 'I want to know what I'm dealing with.' And so that's when I went to get tested. And, and, you know, I don't regret it." As we see in chapter 2, women often decide to get tested so that they can, as Myriad describes, save their own lives and their family.

The idea behind Myriad's BRAC*Analysis* Awareness Campaign was to position Myriad as a company that enables consumers to control their genetic destiny. The company used messaging from a pilot advertising campaign in 2002 that presented BRAC*Analysis* as "a blood test that's helped thousands of women find their risk for hereditary breast and ovarian cancer," thus supplying these women with the tools for empowerment in their medical decisions (Williams-Jones 2006). The test's commercial name is short for its slogan: Be Ready Against Cancer. Overall, though, the campaign is flawed. It simplifies a complex issue, and some of its slogans, such as "reduce my cancer risk now," heighten consumer fear and anxiety and offer false hope by suggesting that the test is a cure for cancer. Once a woman takes the test and learns her BRCA status however, Myriad offers her no further steps of how to medically reduce one's risk.

A study of websites that advertise genetic testing shows that the most common emotional appeals used alongside empowerment were fear and the sadness, guilt, and regret associated with the decision *not* to take the test (Liu & Pearson 2008). Direct-to-consumer genetic testing websites used the theme of empowerment 90 percent of the time as an emotionally persuasive marketing device. Apparently for a woman to be empowered, she simply has to take a test.

Myriad's 2007 advertising campaign used several marketing strategies to increase the consumer market share for the BRAC*Analysis* test. The first of these strategies was to mention only the benefits of consumer genetic testing, often misrepresenting these benefits, while downplaying any negative consequences (Williams 2007). For example, Myriad doesn't mention that some people might suffer employment or insurance discrimination, emotional or psychological damages, negative reactions from family, or, most notably, confusion and uncertainty, if testing gives a false positive, negative, or an ambiguous answer. Dr. Kenneth Offit, a medical oncologist at Memorial Sloan-Kettering Cancer Center in New York, has noted that, in fact, those women who get tested for high-risk mutations such as BRCA are especially vulnerable to getting inconclusive readings. These results can cause even greater distress. He goes on to note:

> We see the same negative effects in women tested for the BRCA genes who were given ambiguous results, as those seen in patients in the early 1990s who received ambiguous test results for Huntington disease. Women with such results, such as missense mutations or "variants of unknown significance," often experienced more upset than those testing either positive or negative for a known mutation." (Brower 2010)

Unlike advertisements for prescription medications, which must list all possible side effects and harms, genetic testing ads do no such thing. And, although it's positive to think that knowledge is power, Myriad does little to suggest the next steps consumers might take once they know that they are, in fact, BRCA mutation carriers. Furthermore, the surprising truth is that a link between genetic testing and cancer prevention has not been proven. Testing companies still make these claims without validation from clinical research studies. A 2005 federal report concluded that various interventions offered to BRCA-positive women—namely, prophylactic mastectomy and oophorectomy—will, in the long run, reduce women's mortality. However, it cautions that most studies conducted on women who elected these preventive measures considered whether they would developed breast cancer rather than whether the women would die from the disease (Nelson et al. 2005). Genetic testing for a high-risk woman can lead to a more informed decision on what to do next—such as more frequent screening or preventive surgery. But the cancer cure touted by genetic testing companies is not actually connected to a reduction in breast and ovarian cancers or in patient mortality (Nelson et al. 2005). The studies did demonstrate some behavioral or psychological benefits of genetic testing—such as decreased levels of distress—yet it also exemplified that while getting tested and subsequent preventative surgery lead to a reduction in *getting cancer*, the study found no corollary between utilizing the genetic test and *preventing death* (Nelson et al. 2005).

A follow-up recommendation upon the 2005 study stated that the evidence on mortality rates remains incomplete and insufficient, which causes difficulty in drawing large conclusions from the data. This is especially true considering the wide range of variants in women's BRCA testing experiences and demographics. In fact, there appears to be a wide variation of breast cancer risk itself among BRCA1/2 mutation carriers. A study in 2008 noted that the standard risk assessment information of BRCA1/2 given out by genetics and on cancer websites uses a single standard set of risk percentages (Begg et al. 2008). However, there appears to be a *wider variation among BRCA carriers* that has neither been widely researched, nor discussed in risk assessment literature. Begg and his colleagues (2008), using population-based cancer registry data between 1985 and 2000, note the presence of multiple risk factors for breast cancer—such as a family history of young women diagnoses, a presence of cancer in both breasts, or a clustering of breast cancer—can increase one's risk of BRCA1/2, while the absence of such factors may lower one's assessment.

Thus, the "cure" of genetic testing and preventative surgery is oftentimes not the best course of action for BRCA-positive mutation women, especially for young women. A recent study on medical decision making in response to a risk of BRCA mutation has estimated that the probability of living to the age of seventy without any interventionist treatment was 53 percent for those carrying the BRCA1 gene, and 71 percent for the carrying the BRCA2 gene (Kurian, Sigal, and Plevritis 2010). To put this in perspective, the probability of those without any BRCA mutation living to age seventy is 84 percent (Kurian, Sigal, and Plevritis 2010). While this study stated that the single most effective intervention choice was a prophylactic oophorectomy by age forty, it described the best combination was a prophylactic mastectomy at twenty-five, and a prophylactic oophorectomy at age forty (Kurian, Sigal, and Plevritis 2010). This means that having preventive surgery around forty years of age provides the best rate of BRCA survival compared to surgeries at much younger ages, and significantly that the age at which women have these surgeries done has a fundamental effect upon their effectiveness, and upon the possibilities of negative side effects.

Ultimately, the report concluded, "although [prophylactic mastectomy] at age 25 plus [prophylactic oophorectomy] at age 40 years maximizes survival probability, substituting mammography plus MRI screening for [pro-phylactic mastectomy] seems to offer comparable survival" (Kurian, Sigal, and Plevritis 2010, 222). Thus, the decision to choose surveillance, including long-term surveillance to screen for possible cancerous cells, rather than immediately scheduled surgeries upon learning one is BRCA positive, can have positive medical effects, in addition to changes this causes to surgeries' financial and physical side effects, and some of these preventative surgeries may well be unnecessary.

Research has shown that even when consumers arrange for testing through their primary physicians, wrong interpretations of genetic testing results can lead to misdiagnosis and unnecessary surgeries (Brierly et al. 2010). These findings are more worrisome because Myriad is currently marketing BRAC*Analysis* to general practitioners, many of whom have little direct experience in treating cancer patients or in genetic counseling. And though Myriad does provide marketing materials to these physicians, such cursory information does not adequately replace expert training in genetics counseling or in the multifaceted interpretation of BRAC*Analysis* results (Brierly et al. 2010).

One woman I spoke with had difficulty first obtaining the test and then finding a health-care professional to discuss its results, her risk, and next steps. Rachel had been asking for the BRCA test for years, and after finally switching doctors, she was able to get it. She describes how she came to be tested.

> I was sitting in the waiting room waiting for the doctor to come in, and I saw a poster on the wall for BRCA analysis. And so, when I went back in, I said, "You know, I've been asking for this test for seven years and my OBGYN wouldn't test me. But you guys offer the test." And she said yes. And I said, "Can I have it today?" And she said yes, and she drew my blood.

At first, Rachel received "some really incorrect information" about her test results. A medical assistant informed her about her risks for both breast and ovarian cancer but she later realized the information was not "actually accurate." She then tried to see her oncologist but was turned away because the oncologist was "too backed up with cancer patients to see someone who didn't have cancer." So, even though Myriad had marketed the test through a doctor's office and that office was willing to order it, no one was able to provide her the best information and support to deal with the results. Her husband ended up calling the Myriad hotline, and company employees put Rachel in touch with "a genetic counselor that works for them who actually gave me correct information." She also got a list of doctors in her area who would arrange for this testing and the website of a support group. Although Rachel's situation got resolved, at first the combination of poorly trained or busy doctors left her without support. Myriad's direct-to-consumer strategy (a poster and hotline) had positioned them as the primary source of "correct" information about the BRCA test results instead of the medical providers closest to Rachel and most familiar with her history and situation.

Direct-to-consumer marketing of genetic testing has grown with the larger medical trend of providing health information and tools to consumers themselves as a means of patient self-empowerment. Consumers are now expected to be proactive for their health and their family's health. This empowerment is an important health initiative. Yet eliminating the healthcare provider from the genetic testing equation leaves consumers without the benefit of medical experts who know the individual being tested. An experienced provider might be able to interpret the genetic results more accurately or in a way that is customized for each patient, and then provide further steps, especially if the results are positive and indicate a predisposition for a given disease.

A lack of expert advice and other factors makes women who test positive for the BRCA mutation overestimate their risk for cancer (Howard, Balneaves, and Bottorff 2009). This has big implications, because a woman's perceived risk influences her testing and treatment decisions more than her actual medical risk (Pilarski 2009). BRCA-positive women often have a sense of genetic determinism—thinking that one gene can accurately predict their future. They describe their bodies as a "ticking time bomb" ready to detonate at any moment. Many seek to eliminate the parts of their bodies that they perceive to be susceptible to cancer. They say that the decision to get mastectomies was a "no-brainer" because they just wanted to "get them off." Some women even expressed the feeling that they "couldn't get [their] ovaries out fast enough." Some describe the BRCA diagnosis as a "huge bomb that just went off in the whole family." The use of such language shows that women come to see parts of their bodies as militaristic devices that have turned against them.

In part, women think this way because they see genetic testing as accurate—they feel they have a 100 percent risk of eventually getting cancer. Having this fatal sense of destiny makes a woman more likely to get preventive surgery, which may be unwarranted given her statistical medical risk.

Such drastic measures make Myriad's advertising profitable to the medical field beyond just genetics testing (Howard, Balneaves, and Bottorff 2009; Tambor, Rimer, and Strigo 1997). Besides, Myriad's health-prevention message fits within the medical model of disease prevention, a model based on risk management, screening, and prevention procedures, and one that is already supported by medical administrators and health-care providers (White et al. 2008; Gold and Carbone 2010).

More than Myriad and its genetic testing counterparts are crucial stakeholders in the genetic testing industry. The physicians who lament the extent of overmedicalization also have a role in it, as well as a share of its profits (Rosenberg 2009). There are numerous professions that rely on genetic testing to ensure a paycheck and employment in both the public and private sectors, from genetic counselors to companies that provide biotechnology production, biochemistry research, and product development and delivery (Holtzman and Watson 1997). Public health workers and health-care providers have also come to support and depend on risk management and preventive models (Rosenberg 2009).

What Does BRCA Advertising Look Like?

As I noted, a lack of research on the link between testing, cancer prevention, and death hasn't kept genetic testing companies from portraying genetic testing as the "cure" for cancer (Gold and Carbone 2010). For example, Cancer Risk Assessment, a company that markets the test OncoVue, which is used to determine hereditary breast cancer risk, says in their advertisements that "early detection is the key to breast cancer survival" and features images of grinning, confident women. The company's slogan for OncoVue is "Beating the odds on Breast Cancer!" (Cancer Risk Assessment 2010). Nowhere on their website, however, does the company explain that getting a false negative, a false positive, or an ambiguous result is possible. Also, despite the company's claim that OncoVue is crucial to beating breast cancer, the website lists very little information about the next steps women who do have a "high risk" should take.

A major selling point for genetic testing companies is empowerment. The idea of taking control of your health is especially appealing to people who feel powerless and scared in the face of the possibility—or what they perceive as the high probability—of being BRCA positive. Pathway Genomics ran an ad for "Affordable Home DNA Testing for health conditions," which depicts

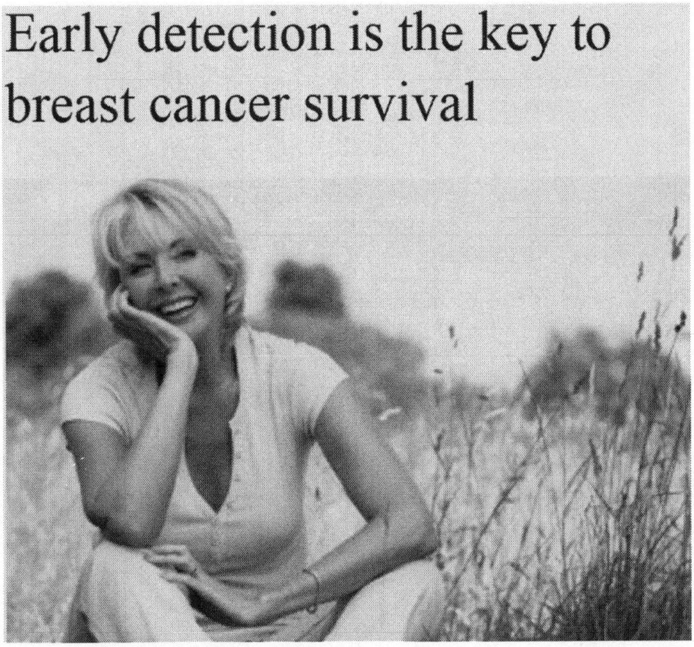

Fig. 1. Retrieved from Cancer Risk Assessment. "About Us." Cancer Risk Assessment. www.cancerriskassessment.com.

a woman dressed in an all-white running outfit joyously running down the beach, seemingly thrilled at using genetic testing to "take control" of her fears about her genetic susceptibility to disease (O'Connor 2010).

Other ads, and even companies' slogans, are no different. The very slogan of Matrix Genomics is "empowering people through genetic knowledge." Yet, like many similar companies, Matrix Genomics offers little substantial advice on how to process and use this "genetic knowledge" once it is obtained. Instead, the ads encourage women to think they can take control of their health simply by taking the genetic test. And the companies provide them with no further resources or steps to continue this medical self-empowerment. What research we have on Americans' perceptions about genetic testing shows that most people are familiar with genetics and have a highly favorable attitude to testing across the board because it gives them control over their health (Condit 2010). Evidently, the messages of Myriad and similar genetic testing companies are beginning to stick.

Genetic testing advertisements convey another emotional message, one

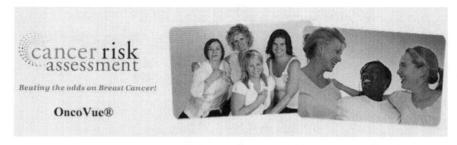

Fig. 2. Retrieved from Cancer Risk Assessment. "About Us." Cancer Risk
Assessment. www.cancerriskassessment.com.

that has many names. Basically, the ads tell women to be terrified by cancer.
It is a message that taps into a deep fear, one that motivates action. This fear
is sometimes called "cancer fatalism," which is the belief that "cancer is a
death sentence" (Hall et al. 2008, 1321). It's also called "cancerphobia," a fear
of cancer that, over half a century ago, surgeon George Crile described as
"more suffering than cancer itself" (Aronowitz 2010, 1431). Genetic testing
companies take advantage of women's fear of cancer, often by linking the
fate of women who have already gotten cancer to their decision not to get
tested. They're telling women: *if you don't get tested, look what could happen to
you*. And they design their message to particularly target women who have a
family history of breast cancer.

Medical ethics professor Dr. Audrey Chapman, who researched the
themes depicted in Myriad's advertising campaign in 2007, points to perhaps the most vivid of these fear tactics. In the playbill for *Wit*, a play based
on the life of a female professor dying from ovarian cancer, Myriad placed
a full-page advertisement showing a woman who clutches her chest with
fear and foreboding. The ad's headline reads: "The only thing worse than
HEARING you have CANCER is hearing it TWICE" (Hull and Prasad
2001). These tactics skillfully connect not getting tested to definitely getting
cancer. And they draw in all women, both those vulnerable because of their
families' medical histories and those who have less reason to worry about
inherited cancer.

The advertisement asks the reader, "If you could discover your risk for
a second breast cancer or for ovarian cancer, would you? Chances are, you
would. . . . Such is the promise of [this test]. . . . Knowing your family history is neither enough, nor is [it] always accurate. [This test] is" (Hull and
Prasad 2001). Such a statement is only relevant to the small percentage of

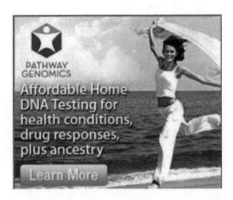

Fig. 3. Retrieved from Shelia O'Connor, "Top News: Walgreens Postpones Carrying Genetic Test Kit." Examiner.com. http://www.examiner.com/sf-in-san-francisco/top-news-walgreens-postpones-carrying-genetic-test-kit-photos.

women who have the BRCA mutation, which is 1 in 200–400 women (Lerman et al. 1995). But it's going out to an entire population of women, and most of them don't need the test. It says to all women diagnosed with breast cancer that taking the test will allow them to discover their risk of getting breast cancer. But really, the test will tell them only whether they have the BRCA mutation or not. Further, it wrongly states that the test is "always accurate," ignoring the possibility of a false negative, a false positive, or an ambiguous result. The ad not only manipulates women to act quickly and "get tested" but also convinces them to act independently of medical advice. The ad suggests that they consult Myriad directly as opposed to consulting a physician.

Another ad using similar fear tactics was published by Myriad in 2001. It shows a young woman nervously wringing her neck (Bowen, Battuello, and Raats 2005). Around her are the phrases "She was told not to worry about breast cancer. . . . Unfortunately she'll be diagnosed next year" (Bowen, Battuello, and Raats 2005). This headline strikes fear into the heart of any woman. The ad implies that all women who come across it are deeply in danger of having breast cancer, even though they think they are healthy. Yet the average woman in her forties (and the woman pictured looks much younger than forty) has a risk of 1.6 percent (Bowen, Battuello, and Raats 2005). The ad then goes on to claim that "Traditional means of assessing risk of sporadic breast cancer fail to identify women with hereditary risk," evidently ignoring the fact that the traditional approach does consider a

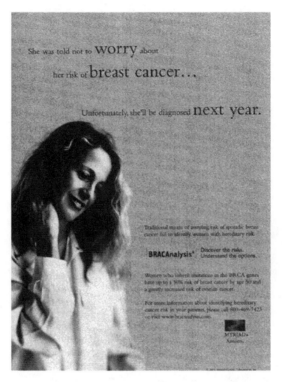

Fig. 4. Retrieved from Deborah J. Bowen, Kathryn M. Battuello, and Monique Raats. 2005. "Marketing Genetic Tests: Empowerment or Snake Oil?" *Health Education & Behavior* 32(5): 676–85. Located on page 680.

woman's family history of cancer, which remains the most reliable indicator of the disease (National Cancer Institute 2012).

The fear evoked by these advertisements seeped into the mass media, which amplified the issue with emotionally charged coverage. One ABC news story, "Split Realities for Sisters with Breast Cancer Gene," used the power of two women's testimonies to show, in vivid detail, how significantly the fear of getting cancer affects women's lives (Pinto 2007). The story covers the experiences of two sisters who both have a high risk for the breast cancer mutation (given their family history) and have tested positive for the BRCA gene (Pinto 2007). One sister decides to have a double mastectomy upon hearing her test results, while the other does not. The article paints a black-and-white picture of the two women. The one who chose the surgical option was "cured" of cancer. The other, who chose not to have surgery,

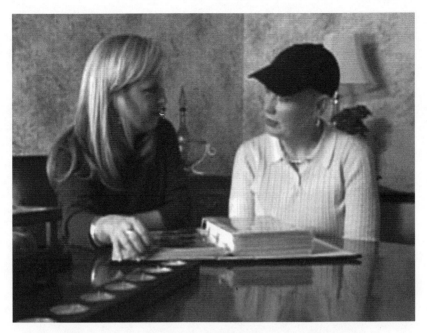

Fig. 5. Retrieved from Barbara Pinto, "Split Realities for Sisters with Breast Cancer Gene." *ABC World News*, October 8, 2007. http://a.abcnews.com/WN/OnCallPlus/story?id=3704741&page=1.

was diagnosed with cancer and, thereafter, has lived in constant fear of her cancer returning.

Such portrayals create a stark ultimatum between preventive surgery and cancer, and they fuel the misconceptions surrounding the BRCA gene. They promote the preventive surgical option by reinforcing the message that testing positive for BRCA1 or BRCA2 undoubtedly means you will get cancer. Little substantial data are provided in the ABC story with regard to the odds of developing breast cancer once a positive diagnosis is given. More than this, the story presupposes that, if a woman waits on a surgical option, she is to blame for developing breast cancer. The sister who did choose to wait points to her sister and notes, "Here's the preventive maintenance." She then points her finger to herself and states, "Here's somebody that held off, and the bomb blew up." The narrative of this "troubling legacy" and the very language of the article provide the reader with faulty information and reinforce the fear of cancer.

Pinto's article goes even further. It talks about how the sisters, upon learning they were BRCA2 positive, were "faced with the painful choice to consider having a mastectomy to avoid breast cancer." This statement frames surgery as the only "cure" for cancer, even though it cannot completely eradicate risk (Bermejo-Perez, Márquez-Calderón, and Llanos-Méndez 2007). The sister who chose surveillance reinforces this erroneous belief: "For the rest of my life, I have to think . . . is the cancer back? That's what I have to think about all the time. [My sister] doesn't have to think about that, but I will" (Pinto 2007). In a way, she is right. Her sister does not have to think about whether cancer will return—but she does have to think about whether she, too, will develop the disease in the breast tissue left behind after her preventive surgery and, perhaps, about how that surgery has damaged some aspects of her life. But the media presents this story as a cautionary tale for all women, even though a substantial minority of BRCA-positive-mutation women will choose to live a fulfilling life without surgery (Litton et al. 2009). The general bias against presenting this nonsurgical option is part of the cancer fatalism that genetic testing companies promote, insinuating that death will come unless you take their genetic test.

A further theme in genetic testing advertising is women's moral obligation to get tested, especially if there is a strong history of cancer in the family. After all, the argument goes, women who are tested can inform other family members who may also be at risk. Companies encourage the sharing of test results between family members, which can draw unwilling persons into the genetic testing network (Van Riper 2005; Van Riper and Gallo 2005). One woman I spoke with suggests that women who test positive may internalize this need to share their test results and encourage unwilling family members to get tested. She says she has been "nagging" her brother "for three or four years to get tested. He has . . . two sons and two daughters." After telling me her brother hasn't been tested yet, she notes, "I think I'm going to have to nag him some more." Advertisements that encourage personal responsibility can result, as in this case, in BRCA-positive individuals dragging family members who would not otherwise be tested into the testing process.

Women who are emotionally estranged from their relatives struggle especially when deciding whether to approach family members with the potentially upsetting news of a BRCA test result (Douglas, Hamilton, and Grubs 2009). Generally, those who are tested reveal the result—whatever it may be—to at least one relative, but further disclosures often are planned in advance or omit certain information to avoid alarming a relative of doing emotional damage (Daly et al. 2001; McGivern et al. 2004; Patenaude et

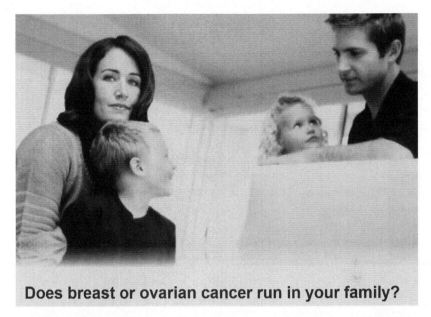

Does breast or ovarian cancer run in your family?

Fig. 6. Retrieved from Myriad Genetics, Inc. "BRACAnalysis." Myriad Genetics. www.bracnow.com.

al. 2006). Although women can have positive experiences with family support, family relationships can also weaken when opinions on test taking and post-testing decision-making differ. Studies show that disclosure can result in isolation and stigmatization (Douglas et al. 2009). So although moral obligation is an effective marketing tool for genetic testing agencies, these companies rarely acknowledge the potential harms of disclosing to family members, nor do they always offer resources to help women fulfill their "obligation."

In another of Myriad's advertisements, a woman is depicted with her husband and two children. As the young daughter looks innocently and helplessly up at her father, who meets his son's laughing gaze, the mother looks worriedly off camera, away from the family group. Underneath the image are the words "Does breast or ovarian cancer run in your family?" (Myriad Genetics 2010). The message conveys a mother worried for her children's sake even more than for her own. It pushes her to test not so much for her own sake but in order to care for her family. On another page of Myriad's website, a testimonial from a woman named Cathy explains to the reader that "Genetic testing helped me . . . do everything in my power to fight the high risk of cancer that runs in my family," yet the website provides little substantial information on how to reduce the risk of breast cancer beyond what physicians and family practitioners recommend (Cathy 2012).

In order to convey the message of moral obligation properly, however, advertisements must also reinforce genetic determinism. Specifically, in the context of BRAC*Analysis* testing, the marketing enforces the message that, if someone in a woman's family had breast cancer, then, undoubtedly, each woman in the hereditary line should fear getting this cancer enough to be tested, not only for herself but to protect her children. In one of Matrix Genomics' online advertisements, a photograph shows a young woman between two older women, presumably her mother and her aunt. Beneath their grinning faces the advertisement reads, "You inherited your grandmother's sense of humor. Do you also share her susceptibility to breast cancer?" (Matrix Genomics 2012). This image reinforces the message that if a woman has breast cancer, every member of her family is likely to have cancer as well. Another image on the Matrix Genomics website, in this case addressing Alzheimer's disease, features four generations of women with bright blue eyes. It asks, "So you got your grandmother's eyes. Did you also inherit her tendency toward Alzheimer's Disease?" (Matrix Genomics 2012). This ad has a stronger effect than the one about breast cancer because it implies that the genetic risk of Alzheimer's has definitely been inherited and confirmed, as has the genetic legacy of blue eyes. All the females *have* inherited the elder woman's eye color; inheriting a sense of humor through genetics is more of a stretch. Still, these advertisements not only strike fear in the heart of any woman whose family has had a history of breast cancer or Alzheimer's but also encourage repeated and expensive testing within the family.

Another women I spoke with, Dana, described the role of Myriad's DTC campaign in her own BRCA-testing experience. She first learned about the test because her aunt tested positive and encouraged her and her sister to get tested as well. "She wasn't trying to force us," Dana recalls. "She didn't even . . . communicate with us verbally. She just . . . sent us emails." In these messages, she mentioned her positive result and provided a list of genetic counselors in the area in case Dana and her sister were interested in testing. More interesting is another way Dana's aunt approached the topic.

> She sent us all this informational material from Myriad Laboratory, like a little packet that they had put together for women to send . . . to share with their relatives their positive statuses. So she sent us all of Myriad's informational packet that was already predesigned for this situation.

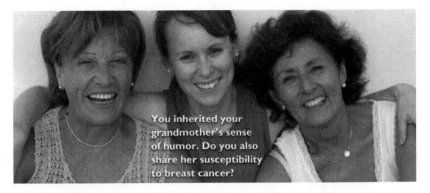

You inherited your grandmother's sense of humor. Do you also share her susceptibility to breast cancer?

Fig. 7. Retrieved from Matrix Genomics. "Personal Genomics to Enhance your Life and Life Expectancy!" Matrix Genomics. http://www.matrixgenomics.com/index.php.

Dana heard about the test through her aunt, but her aunt was armed with information from Myriad, which is both marketing familial responsibility and, by reaching consumers directly through their relatives, bypassing the medical experts who are trained to provide accurate and individualized counseling about the risks of hereditary diseases. In this way, Myriad takes advantage of BRCA-positive women in order to reach additional consumers.

Research suggests that Myriad's advertising campaign has paid off economically. Estimates are that, because of its DTC advertising, Myriad experienced a "244% increase in referrals for genetic services compared with the year before the campaign. The advertising campaign also led to an increased interest in genetic services by women who were at lower risk for being mutation carriers" (Leachman et al. 2011, 36). Less than one month into its 2007 campaign, Myriad's stock went through the roof. Its revenue increased by 55 percent and gross profits by 70 percent (Myriad Genetics 2007). Even its 2002 pilot advertising campaign in Atlanta and Denver led to higher rates of medical consumers requesting BRCA*Analysis*, yet reports also concluded that health-care providers were not prepared with adequate information or resources to advise their patients on the BRCA1 and BRCA2 gene mutations or on whether genetic testing was relevant for their patients (Williams-Jones 2006).

Consumer interest continues to grow and is reflected in Myriad's increasing revenue: its third fiscal quarter, which ended on March 31, 2011, was its best to date, with a 13 percent increase in revenue, from $90.8 million in the same quarter of 2010 to $102.4 million in 2011. Fiscal second-quarter earnings rose 17 percent according to a January 2012 report. As Myriad's presi-

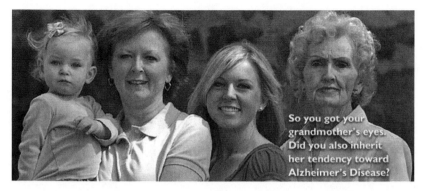

So you got your
grandmother's eyes.
Did you also inherit
her tendency toward
Alzheimer's Disease?

Fig. 8. Retrieved from Matrix Genomics. "Personal Genomics to Enhance your Life and Life Expectancy!" Matrix Genomics. http://www.matrixgenomics.com/index.php.

dent, Peter D. Meldrum, states, "We delivered the best revenue and operating income results for any quarter in our history" (Myriad Genetics 2011). The BRAC*Analysis* test specifically is gaining in popularity and profitability. Total revenue for this test in the second quarter of 2012 was $101.4 million, a 14 percent increase over the same period of the prior year (Myriad Genetics 2012). Revenue for this test was $90.3 million in the third fiscal quarter of 2011, up from $79.8 million in 2010 (Myriad Genetics 2011). Evidently, Myriad's advertising campaigns have given a huge boost to the test's profitability. Considering, however, that the price of the test has been consistently increasing as the cost of the company's genetic research has been steadily decreasing, Myriad appears to be more concerned with turning a profit than with raising awareness of hereditary breast cancer (Matloff and Caplan 2008; Yale Cancer Genetic Counseling 2010).

Given the money made from Myriad's DTC marketing of BRAC*Analysis* testing, Pathway Genomics designed a similar marketing campaign to advertise a genetic test touted to discover, among other things, gene mutations indicating an increased risk for breast cancer. However, its plan to sell these tests at Walgreens stores nationwide prompted the FDA to block the marketing of this test. Currently, the FDA is investigating several genetic testing companies and recently warned companies such as American International Biotechnology Services, Lumigenix, and Precision Quality DNA that their DTC genetic testing services may need to be reviewed and approved (Vorhaus 2011). As of the summer of 2011, the FDA has sent twenty-three such warning letters and is now requiring DTC companies to back up the advertising claims made on their websites (Vorhaus 2011). The FDA has yet to determine the specific aspects of the industry that should be regulated in order to protect consumers and just how to assess the claims of genetic tests. Causing further confusion is the reality that there is no internationally agreed-upon definition of genetic testing, as it remains a new field of medical study (Hogarth, Javitt, and Melzer 2008). As we have seen, many factors are allowing the genetic testing industry to continue to grow; so, in order to address genetic testing in the United States fully, the FDA may need more time and resources than are available today.

The FDA has taken insufficient steps so far to consider how to best regulate the complex and rapidly changing world of DTC genetic testing and marketing. And it has had some time to grapple with this issue, although genetic testing is relatively new. After all, there have been calls for regulation and reform since Myriad first began marketing its genetic testing products in 1999 (Bowen, Battuello, and Raats 2005). A first step would be to determine whether the genetic testing kits provided directly to consumers (without the intervention of a medical provider) are truly needed. Also, meeting consumer demand must not bar the creation of guidelines for these tests, although to date few, if any, regulations are in place. Standards for determining the efficacy of genetic testing kits, as well as for defining what constitutes genetic testing, need to be nationally agreed upon. If genetic testing kits are deemed to be medically appropriate and effective, then the second step of increased regulation must concern the products' marketing. FDA control over genetic testing must be equal to the control it exerts over prescription medication; genetic testing companies must advertise the potential benefits as well as the potential drawbacks of their products in order to provide consumers with unbiased and accurate information (Gollust, Hull, and Wilfond 2002). It remains to be seen how private companies working for a profit (i.e., Myriad and similar companies) will cooperate with public institutions dedicated to improving national health care.

I've Got a Test for You: The Normalization of Genetic Testing

Scholars, and in particular, sociologists, have been heavily involved in researching how genetic knowledge is constructed (Atkinson 1997; Conrad and Gabe 1999). Early on, social science researchers specifically addressed the historical emergence and social implications of new technologies—such as genetic testing—as well as the potential control and power implications that come with "new genetic knowledge regimes" that frame genetic risk and the dissemination of genetic testing information (Foucault 1991; Atkinson 1997; Atkinson and Glasner 2007; Atkinson, Glasner, and Lock 2009; Conrad and Gabe 1999; Armstrong 1995; Aronowitz 2009). Early feminist researchers focused specifically on breast cancer diagnoses and the social construction of this disease and its treatments, by drawing on a range of feminist approaches across a variety of disciplines, including media studies, bioethics, psychology, and sociology (Potts 2000).

When it comes to testing for BRCA, women (and men) are faced not only with making decisions about genetic testing in a complex and relatively unregulated market in which companies are pursuing vigorous direct-to-consumer ad campaigns but also with evaluating the claims of an expanding number of genetic testing labs and biotech companies. As Browner and Preloran note, "Whereas in 1997 there were 332 labs and biotech companies engaged in the development or clinical use of genetic tests, by 2009 there were 603 labs testing for 1,715 different genetic diseases" (Browner and Preloran 2010, 117). This growth has normalized genetic testing. It has become a part of standard health care.

The commercialization of genetic testing has created a new "bio-economy" that is rapidly becoming corporatized (Martin 1995; Clarke et al. 2003). The selling of genetic information constitutes an increasingly profitable sector of our economy, as profits from "bio-wealth" continue to expand. If you want proof, check out the financial revenues of genetic testing agencies. Of even greater concern than the expansion of the bio-economy, however, is that more and more aspects of public health care are being patented and commoditized. Corporations are using public health data to generate private profit (Clarke et al. 2003; Clarke et al. 2010). As genetic testing for a range of chronic diseases grows, so does the perception that a large majority of the population is living in a high-risk state for developing a life-threatening or chronic illness.

By the fall of 2007, genetic testing companies began providing consumers with the opportunity to purchase a genome scan directly online—without the authorization of a physician. Two companies—deCODEme, from Reykjavik, Iceland, and 23andMe, in Mountain View, California—began charging $1,000 per customer for a genome scan. And the process is easy. You only have to provide saliva in a tube for genetic analysis in order to have your DNA scanned for a wide variety of genetic risks such as Alzheimer's disease, heart disease, multiple sclerosis, and prostrate cancer. You can even access your results easily, via the company's secure website. And this is only the beginning of where genetic testing can lead.

Genetic testing continues to gain consumer attention. For example, 23andMe's commercial genetic test was named invention of the year by *Time* magazine in 2008 for "pioneering retail genomics." 23andMe also compiles client's genetic information into a huge database to contribute to research in the field of genetic medicine.23andMe has created online groups, so individuals can share and compare their personal genetic information, and it is becoming increasingly common for parents to be to choose genes for their baby deliberately (Clarke et al. 2003; Lee 2009). These developments indicate that genetic testing is becoming normalized, even though it is still not adequately regulated.

Research into the efficacy of commercial genetic testing kits reveals that there is little quality control over the types of marketed kits. Also, as discussed, the FDA does not adequately ensure the legitimacy of the promises made by the genetic testing industry concerning the efficacy of these kits (Liu and Pearson 2008). It is ultimately the consumer who decides whether a test will be useful, and, as demonstrated, false advertising often significantly influences these decisions (Hogarth, Javitt, and Melzer 2008). Once someone receives a test result, the statistical risks provided for either a positive or negative result are usually based on statistical models of disease using very limited and nondiverse samples of the population. So, given the unregulated nature of the DTC testing industry, how can a consumer properly interpret a given test result? And what should be done about her or his risk, once the test result is interpreted? Furthermore, the FDA does not regulate the content of advertising or communication from the genetic testing agencies to the consumer, so the consumer has no idea whether the information from the company on his or her risk level is actually correct (Liu and Pearson 2008). The rapid development of DTC genetic testing further complicates the efforts to regulate this industry, especially with regard to the ethical and psychological implications of these tests for the consumer. Although genetic information may be important in the prevention of illnesses, especially in the prevention of chronic disorders, the revelation of genetic risk remains problematic; it is difficult to translate such test results to health prevention, especially when the health-care providers' expertise is not included in the typical genetic testing model.

Although DTC testing can pave the way for some people (consumers) to engage in proactive and preventive health-promoting behaviors based on their genetic results, research on the actual benefits accrued from the increased use of prevention strategies is sparse. For example, BRCA-positive women may decide to have regular screenings for breast cancer. But does this translate into fewer breast cancer deaths or better treatment for those diagnosed with the disease? Although recent evidence suggests that preventive surgeries such as mastectomies and oophorectomies significantly reduce the risks of breast and ovarian cancers, as well as cancer-specific and all-cause mortality, the question remains: when should we begin taking preventive action? (Pruthi, Gostout, and Lindor 2010). When does prevention start too soon? Should we be as worried about precancer as we are about cancer? The link between genetic susceptibility and prevention is, in the words of one scientist, a "promissory science," one that holds out hope that, once we know our genetic makeup, we can, in fact, prevent potentially life-threatening illness (Hedgecoe 2011). But how likely are these promises to come true?

One of the consequences of the normalization and proliferation of genetic testing is that many people may begin to take on new somatic identities; they may come to view their bodies as at risk for a range of diseases (Clarke et al. 2003). Living with this genetic knowledge may not give them the power to do something to head off future health problems, especially when these tests cannot guarantee whether or not someone will develop a certain genetic disorder. Getting tested can also put individuals in a state of "pre-disease," a state of limbo between not having the disease and continually fearing its onset down the road. People living in this pre-disease state provide a growing market for technologies that will further prevent genetic disorders from surfacing, including screening, preventive surgeries, and further medical testing. Because of cancerphobia, consumer anxiety, and the advertising of genetic testing as a "cure," women are increasingly being tested and found positive for the BRCA mutation. Then they seem to enter an uncertain world, as they wait for the cancer to appear in their bodies and listen to the various and confusing voices telling them what they should do to avoid their genetic "destiny." In the meantime, these young women must still try to continue their lives, and they often consider preventive surgeries, especially oophorectomies, to prevent cancer. The desire to have surgery is often so great that young women feel pressure to find a boyfriend, get married, and have children in order to remove their reproductive organs that much sooner (Lydersen 2010; Werner-Lin 2008).

Another concern raised by the current testing model is that, by focusing on genes as the culprit of disease, people ignore the other factors that may play more critical roles in the development of life-threatening and chronic disorders. For example, environmental toxins produced by commercial chemical and manufacturing industries continue to pollute our water and air, and these contribute to the growth of disease, perhaps even more so than the population's genetic makeup (North and Martin 2008). Furthermore, these toxins themselves can cause gene mutations.

Unfortunately, the general public, by and large, does not have a good understanding of this gene-environment interaction and continues to neglect the societal and corporate-driven threats to our health and see genetic testing as the "cure" for genetic ailments (Condit 2010). As we continue to look inward for the causes of illness and blame the victim and her genes, we miss a critical and necessary opportunity to look outward for a range of causal environmental, societal, and cultural factors that also need to be addressed.

The implications of the increasing normalization of genetic testing are worrisome as we look to the future of this technology. Currently, more and more medical conditions—both chronic and acute—as well as more and more socially problematic behaviors, such as drug and alcohol addictions, are coming under the surveillance of our testing culture. Lippman (1991) employed the concept of "geneticization" to describe the tendency to categorize specific populations into social groups according to their "good genes" and "bad genes" (15). Similarly, Zola (1974; 1977) coined the term *medicalization* to describe how medical expertise comes to redefine, and then render problematic, a range of human conditions that now become treated as medical issues.

Evidently, we have already begun to narrow our focus to what is defective within ourselves, rather than concentrating on what role the environment and society play in disease promotion. Perhaps the next step along this testing route is the labeling and categorizing of who is "normal" and who is "abnormal," based solely on their genetic makeup. It does not seem unlikely that the strategy of selectively applying genetic engineering as a way to select for only those genes deemed to be "good" will grow rapidly in the near future.

This cataloguing of populations based on genes is not a new idea in human history. The early twentieth century saw the rise of a strong eugenics movement that swept across America and Europe, built on the ideas of nineteenth-century naturalist Charles Darwin, who hypothesized that natural selection could explain how a given species was able to evolve over time in response to an ever-changing natural environment (Darwin [1859] 2003). Others began to apply natural selection to human populations in a philosophy known as Social Darwinism, which touted the idea of the survival of the fittest. The eugenics movement originated partially from this idea. Proponents thought it was possible to improve the human species through regulating its reproduction, promoting the hereditary traits deemed desirable, and reducing the continuation of undesirable traits (Burke and Castaneda 2007). Populations were "cleansed" of their identifiable physical, mental, and social defects through such practices as forced sterilization, euthanasia, and, in some cases, the extermination of entire populations carrying these "undesirable" traits. A horrific example of this ethnic cleansing was the Nazi's mass extermination of Jews and other "undesirable populations" during World War II. Many eugenic practices continued well into the twentieth century; for example, in studies that focused on how race is linked to intelligence and crime (Herrnstein and Murray 1996; Ossorio, Pilar, and Duster 2005). With the growing normalization and proliferation of genetic testing technologies, we have to be vigilant that they are not used for unjust and inhumane purposes.

Women's Experience with the Genetic Testing Industry

As the genetic testing industry grows, so does the population of men and women who are opting for these tests. Yet few have examined the impact of genetic testing on the lives of women who test positive for gene mutations that put them at risk for particular diseases. Some studies conducted over the past few decades provide us with a glimpse of the impact of genetic testing and examine this impact through the eyes of those who have undergone genetic testing. But there is much more to explore. The decision to be tested or not is complex. It is not as simple as getting your blood drawn and taking advantage of the "power of knowledge" that genetic testing agencies are eager to promote. The experiences of women who test positive for the BRCA1 and BRCA2 gene mutations provide a wealth of important information about the impact of genetic testing on the lives of individuals and their families. And these experiences can serve as examples of what is to come, as the pace of genetic testing continues to increase both nationally and globally. The rest of this book shows how diverse these experiences are—and how powerful and moving. It will follow the women who ultimately test positive for the BRCA mutation and convey, in their own words, the story of their journey—from making the decision to get tested to telling their families and making decisions about cancer prevention.

TWO

Ready for the Test

My mom died of breast cancer when she was twenty-six. I was six months old. She was diagnosed when she was pregnant with me. I'm the sixth cancer survivor going back to my grandmother's generation. So, my mom and one of my mom's sisters, and my grandfather had two sisters, and my grandmother had a sister, who all had breast cancer. So, that's what I mean by, like, a really strong, strong family history. When my mom was diagnosed, it was back in 1970, and so, they just had started doing mammograms back then. So, um, so they obviously didn't know anything about a gene. . . . But I did always know of the family history. I always knew that my mom died of breast cancer. It was just something I always knew. From as early, as young as I can remember, I always was aware of that. It scared me because I was always scared that I would end up having breast cancer and then I would die. Um, it definitely made me more aware of mortality. I think, because I was such—'cause I knew about it at such a young age, I thought about it differently, I think, than a lot of other kids. I think I'm a little, still paranoid about people dying around me.

Jennifer is in her mid-thirties and, like many others living out the BRCA experience, she has long known about her cancer risk and bore the burden of a strong family history of breast cancer. Throughout her young life, she was waiting for cancer to come. So why didn't she get tested for the BRCA mutation as soon as she could?

Let's look at her whole story. Despite not knowing her BRCA status, the fear of her own cancer diagnosis burdened her from a young age. She began having mammograms at seventeen. Because she was so young for the procedure, she had to explain her story to care providers each time. Doctors and technicians alike were surprised to see such a young woman coming in for the test. She even struggled to justify the expense to her HMO. When looking for new career opportunities, she was limited to larger employers that offered a PPO with more coverage. What Jennifer viewed as an essential, lifesaving procedure, insurance providers viewed as an extravagant expense.

In her twenties—in the early 1990s—Jennifer finally talked to a genetic counselor about getting tested. But she was persuaded that she was too young for cancer.

> Okay, so in my twenties I think is around the time when they started doing genetic tests. It was really premature. I went and talked to a genetic counselor. And the time, my impression was that, because it was such early, early phase, I guess, of the testing, they're kind of saying, "Well, you know, we can test you, but just because you test negative doesn't mean you don't have it." And for me it was just too much and confusing, and I thought, well, I don't know if it's really worth it. And I almost felt kind of talked out of it, in a way. . . . And that was my early twenties, and I think I just maybe thought of it differently than I did later on. But at the time, it was more because I think my dad was pushing me into looking into it. I did it for different reasons. . . . The other thing was, it was so expensive, my insurance wouldn't cover it at the time. So, it was, even with my history, it was maybe two thousand dollars out-of-pocket and I just couldn't afford it at twenty-one, twenty-two. I just couldn't. And that was actually a huge contributor to why I didn't do it, actually.

Jennifer gave up on getting tested but continued her regular mammograms. After about a decade passed, she developed fibrocystic breasts, they found a lump in her mammogram, and had increasing pain in her breast. She knew cancer had come. And still, despite all the physical issues and her family's extensive history of breast cancer, the breast surgeon thought she was too young to have cancer and explained the lump as a side effect of the birth control pill. To make sure, the surgeon had Jennifer get an ultrasound, which revealed something suspicious. The medical technician who performed the ultrasound was finally able to convince the doctor to go ahead with a biopsy, more testing, and an MRI, which ultimately showed that Jennifer did, in fact, have cancer.

Although some women get tested because of pressure from their doctor, sometimes almost the opposite occurs—as in Jennifer's case. Jennifer didn't actually find out she had the BRCA mutation until after being diagnosed with breast cancer at age thirty-two. Women like Jennifer can spend years trying to convince their doctor to authorize the BRCA test, often because medical providers see women in their twenties as too young to worry about cancer. Even when she had some irregularities in her breasts, Jennifer's doctors did not want to go through with the biopsy and further testing. Without the support of insurance providers and medical professionals, young women often struggle alone to combat their risk for breast cancer.

Why Get Tested?

Women do not always need a test to tell them cancer will come. But sometimes that confirmation—hearing your doctor say the result is positive—can completely change your world. Genetic testing might make women fear more for their future or at least lose confidence in their ability to address it. So why even have that test? I spoke with dozens of women with different stories, but they all had at least one thing in common: they were tested for the BRCA mutation. So how do these many women reach the point of testing? Why do some women choose to be tested as soon as they can while others live with their strong family history of breast and ovarian cancer but wait for years to get tested? As I learned in my interviews, there are many reasons for women to get tested, but one reason rises above the rest: to beat cancer.

I heard over and over that women get tested because they believe the "power of genetic knowledge" will be their front line of defense against cancer and will enable them to change their genetic destiny. One woman knew she needed the test because it would force the ultimate decision about preventive surgery. She said, I can "sit and wait and get cancer, or do something about it." Another woman described the test in terms of the opportunities it gave her that weren't available to her relatives. She told me she could "almost hear" her mother, who died of breast cancer: "She's standing beside me, saying. . . . 'Well do it! Are you crazy? Don't wait to get cancer!'" Genetic testing, especially for those whose insurance can cover the cost, is an opportunity that most women's mothers and grandmothers did not have. In their minds, their loved ones died without the benefit of the "power" or "control" provided by genetic testing and preventive surgeries. Women are grateful and in awe of their ability to obtain the knowledge necessary to make a preemptive strike against cancer and take control of their genetic destiny.

Women are driven by a sense of inevitability. A positive diagnosis, in the words of one woman, meant she had to wonder "not if, but when I will get cancer." Especially for women with a strong history of breast or ovarian cancer in their families, they feel they must be ready either to act on their testing result or suffer the consequences. Some women, though, are not ready to take that action, so instead they delay getting tested for many years. They wait to confirm what they "already knew." And being ready to know depends on a variety of factors, which I discuss in the next section of this chapter.

In many ways, the messages of power and prevention promoted by direct-to-consumer genetics marketing campaigns mirror what women say about their own experiences. Women see genetic testing as the front line against cancer and a way to lessen their fears. Many of the women I spoke with make this link directly, saying, "I don't want to be sick," and "I would not want to be tested unless I could prevent cancer."

Other women are more specific about how the test will benefit their personal lives. One woman was sure she would prevent cancer by having a mastectomy and reconstructive surgery, which, she said, would increase her chances of getting married: "If I have a mastectomy, then I won't have to be single and have chemotherapy and lose my looks." Another woman wants to be tested because, for her, knowledge is power: "I want to know what I'm dealing with . . . [Testing] will give me information that I can act on."

When women are ready to beat cancer, BRCA testing is the answer.

Being Ready

Becoming ready for the test is an incredibly personal process for every woman, but when I spoke with them—ready or not—their stories often overlapped. Several common themes are woven into the testing pathways women take on their BRCA journeys. Unfortunately, some women get tested before they're completely ready. A woman may find herself unprepared to deal with the results, making the experience negative and even harmful to her emotional health and social life. Every woman must come to feel ready in her own time, and when she does, it can even provide a feeling of empowerment in an otherwise helpless situation. BRCA testing puts control back into women's hands; the main reason the women I surveyed gave for getting tested was "to plan for the future." That future may involve preventive screening, treatment, and surgery. When women are ready to face these obstacles, they have reached the right time for the test.

But women who take the BRCA test can be at very different points in their lives. They might be old or young; some get tested with no prior knowledge of their risk, and others have lived for decades with the possibility of cancer, waiting for the right time to get tested. Endless circumstances affect women's testing decisions, including age, children, employment, religion, and ethnicity. What, then, are the common factors in women's stories? What brings these women from different walks of life to decide, ultimately, that this is the right time to get tested? In this section, let's look at some of the personal and logistical factors that make a woman ready for the BRCA test. Then we can dive into women's stories to see how these experiences play out in real women's lives.

Like with many decisions a woman makes in her lifetime, family comes to the fore. Because BRCA is a hereditary disease, a woman must think about her immediate and extended family: Are my children at risk? Will my husband support my decision to be tested? Who else needs to know about my results? Will my test help my family make their own decisions? One study showed that 90 percent of women's most important or only reason for getting tested is to provide genetic knowledge for their family. Many call their decision an "altruistic act" (Hallowell et al. 2003, 76). Sixty percent of the women I surveyed said that telling their family was a very important reason for testing. At the same time, uncertainty about the effect a BRCA-positive status could have on a woman's family is one of main reasons she might hesitate to get tested. A woman wonders, "Will my family be angry if I bring this burden, this knowledge of hereditary cancer to the family?"

And perhaps most importantly, a woman thinks about her mother, or her sister, or her aunt, or whatever relatives she has watched go through breast cancer diagnoses and BRCA testing. Some women are thrown into the test more suddenly, but for most a family history of cancer is crucial to their decision. Fifty-nine percent of the women I surveyed specifically had a mother diagnosed with breast cancer and 83 percent had at least one family member who had been diagnosed as BRCA positive.

Sometimes women who are diagnosed with breast cancer get the BRCA test, even without other cancer diagnoses in their family. Why? Their doctors. A breast or ovarian cancer diagnosis alone prompts some health-care providers to recommend the test. Such an unexpected suggestion and the shock of a BRCA-positive mutation result can be a disempowering experience for women—a doctor's recommendation alone is not enough to make women ready for the results.

One woman in this situation, Diane, got the BRCA test at her doctor's suggestion and was unprepared to deal with the news that she was BRCA positive. Diane had no family history of breast or ovarian cancer whatsoever, so she never even considered herself at risk for cancer, never mind the BRCA mutation. When she got a biopsy after a routine mammogram showed an irregularity, the surgeon also ordered the BRCA test, even though Diane "didn't even really realize what was going on . . . [or] what the BRCA test was." Getting both the BRCA-positive result and a breast cancer diagnosis sent her into shock.

> I didn't want to have to deal with the logical ins and outs. I just—I was just emotionally distraught. And I just didn't want to have to—[I didn't do research online because if I did] it was almost sort of that I would be embracing the fact that I had cancer. So I was like, I hated so bad that I had [the BRCA mutation] that I didn't even want to even acknowledge it. I didn't want to give it a place in my life at all.

A cancer diagnosis is hard enough. But instead of waiting until she was ready to know she is BRCA positive, she "was just doing what the doctors told me to do."

Family also comes into play for the many women who worry about passing the BRCA mutation on to their children. Research shows that women often get tested for their children's sake (Hallowell et al. 2005). My own research findings support this trend: 82 percent of women with children stated that it was "very" or "somewhat important" to have the BRCA test in order to learn about their children's risk. Aspiring mothers also worry about the risk of their planned children, especially young women who have long known of their high cancer risk. One woman who was tested at age twenty-nine said, "The thing that actually made me finally get tested was the fact that I wanted to start a family, and I wanted to know what I was working with." She needed to understand her own risk fully before she could consider having children. Some women do not want to take the chance of passing the BRCA gene on to their children. One research study found that more than 10 percent of women who were at a high risk for the BRCA mutation would actually consider not having children if they were tested positive (Fortuny et al. 2009). Because the influence family has on women's decisions is clearly so extensive, we return to it later in this chapter.

Family is important in some way for every woman, but what about personal beliefs and religion? None of the women I interviewed said religion was "very important" in their decision to be tested, but some certainly considered it. Women with Ashkenazi Jewish backgrounds are especially prone to breast cancer (lifetime risk of 82 percent) because they are at an increased risk for both strains of the BRCA mutation (Mor and Oberle 2008). When deciding about the test, practicing Ashkenazi Jewish women consider the Jewish code of ethics, or Jewish law, as well as how their community will respond to a BRCA-positive mutation diagnosis. Under Jewish law, decision-making is guided by one's obligations and responsibilities to the broader collective, rather than by more personal considerations (see Mozersky 2012). So it is likely that these women may not feel the same degree of individual autonomy as many other women. Jewish law also mandates, however, that a woman may seek knowledge only if she is emotionally able to deal with it; so a woman may not get tested if she feels unready or thinks the test results will harm her. Furthermore, a preventive mastectomy might be interpreted as self-harming (Mor and Oberle 2008).

A few women who spoke with me delved deeper into the influence of an Orthodox Jewish community on when or if a woman decides to be tested.

> A lot of the [Orthodox Jewish] fathers don't, I think don't want their daughters to be tested. . . . Because then they're not as suitable for marriage. And, that's, and I think that's just a fear that they're not going to be able to find a husband for their daughter, and then maybe once their daughter is married, then they might get tested, but maybe it's too late. Maybe they're too old, maybe they already have cancer, and that's how they find out. I think that there's probably a big number of people my age that don't even know they're at risk because their family's not open about it.

Being part of an Orthodox community may lead some of these women away from BRCA testing because of their traditional beliefs about what makes women suitable for marriage.

More so than actively dissuading Jewish women from the BRCA test, an Orthodox community is more likely to not even talk about it. One woman I spoke with had tried and failed to convey the importance of BRCA testing to both an Orthodox branch of her own family and to male rabbis in her local community.

> But then there is a branch in the family, um, and they are Orthodox Jews. And the last I heard, well one of the fathers died of pancreatic. And he did have children, so those children are at very high risk

of potentially having—fifty-fifty, probably. And the other brothers, I don't know if they tested or not. And, um, I, my mom notified them while she was sick, and they were very rude. And I followed up because I felt like it was my mother's wish to make sure that they had their information. And so I appealed to a different part of that branch of the family. And, um, it was just kind of like, you know, at first it wasn't well received and they called me, I think it was like six months or eight months later, to ask me more about the gene. They claimed that nobody had been diagnosed, but I don't know. I don't know why they called me up. I think something happened, you know, so they wanted to know what the mutation was . . .

And actually I reached out also to the Jewish community, the Rabbinical community, because I thought that they would also be helpful in advocating for the Jewish community. And the male rabbis wanted—they just hand, they do not understand. You know, they, they um, I think it's very easy for them at this stage to, um, they're burying their head in the sand, and the guys, that this is a women's issue.

Despite the higher risk of the BRCA mutation among Ashkenazi Jews, none of the women I interviewed identified as Orthodox themselves. Their absence might show that the taboo around testing makes it much less likely among Orthodox communities. Or perhaps that taboo keeps women from openly taking about their BRCA-positive mutation status—particularly with someone from outside the community like me. Either way, one's religious community can clearly impact women's decisions about the BRCA test.

Women feel ready for BRCA testing not only for personal reasons but also practical—especially financial—ones. Women are more likely to be ready if they are financially comfortable and have received at least some college education. To begin with, these women are much more likely to have heard of the BRCA mutation, and, obviously, a woman has to know the genetic testing option exists before she decides to pursue it. Women who are financially comfortable are over four times as likely to be aware of the BRCA mutation than women who are not, and those with some college are over 2.5 times more likely to get tested than those who have only a high school degree (Tambor, Rimer, and Strigo 1997). Systematic economic barriers widen the gap between women who are and are not financially well off. Those with less money tend to lack both health insurance and access to information about the development of genetic testing technology (Tambor, Rimer, and Strigo 1997).

If a woman isn't immediately prepared to pay for the BRCA test and whatever preventive measures may follow, she has to wait. Being financially ready can mean having insurance that covers BRCA testing, having enough money for an expensive surgery, and being able to take time off while recovering from surgery. The substantial cost of the test itself—$3,000–$5,000 depending on wait times and its comprehensiveness—is a big deterrent, especially when some health insurance companies decline to cover it prior to an actual cancer diagnosis. BRCA testing can also affect the entire family's finances. One study revealed that most spouses of women at high risk for the BRCA mutation worried that the test would hurt the family's health insurance coverage (Bluman et al. 2003).

> That was another reason I stayed up at night worrying, because I thought, "How in the world are we going to pay for all of this?" . . . I was trying to pay [Myriad Genetics] a little bit every month, and then they got greedy and wanted more. And I told them that they're welcome to come get my first-born child, but I can't get them any more than what I'm giving them. . . . So I'm still paying that off. I still owe them probably $1,200.

That's how one woman explains the payments left after getting the BRCA test, which her insurance wouldn't fully cover because they claimed that it wasn't medically necessary. And with the combination of surgical and hospital bills at the end of the process, she ended up paying "around $30,000" out of pocket in all. This enormous sum is no doubt impossible for most women to afford and prevents them from getting tested to begin with and taking further preventive steps. A full 64 percent of the women I surveyed said that their worries about losing insurance were a very or somewhat important factor in making them hesitate to get tested. In fact, this worry more than any other factor delayed their decisions to get the test.

An obvious question to ask is how old women are when they decide to get tested. In my study, women got tested, on average, at thirty-six years old. The youngest woman I spoke with was eighteen when she got tested; the eldest was sixty-five. Although older women feel they are in the "right" place in their lives to come to terms with the possibility of a positive result, both elderly and very young women tend to be the least informed about the BRCA mutation gene (Mogilner et al. 1998). Perhaps because of this, or because they think they are too old to benefit from knowing their status, women over the age of sixty tend to be three times less interested in BRCA testing than younger women (Tambor, Rimer, and Strigo 1997; Mogilner et al. 1998).

And how could a woman as young as eighteen be ready for the BRCA test? Interestingly, among the women I surveyed, using online support groups was tied to getting tested at a younger age. I can only speculate as to why. It could merely be a reflection of the fact that younger people are more tech savvy and are more likely to use the Internet to begin with. But it could also show that having information available online helps make them feel ready. When a woman can search "BRCA" online and get thousands of results, she can be well informed and surer about getting tested. If she's one of the first in her family to deal with BRCA testing, she can instead follow the footsteps of the many BRCA-positive women who came before her and who now share their experiences online. Online communities may help a woman become ready for the test more quickly.

Ultimately, women feel ready to get tested when they're ready to take action on our earlier question: why get tested? The testing decision is merely the stepping-stone to prevention. A woman is ready for the test when she's ready to face cancer by getting surgery or more screening. Of the women I talked with, 80 percent said that a very important reason for taking the test was "to make surgery decisions" and 76 percent wanted to know whether they needed "to increase screening." As one woman explained, she initially "had no idea that there was anything you could do proactively . . . to reduce your risk other than the surveillance." Only several years later, when she learned about and was ready for surgery, did she finally get tested. She said, "If I had tested positive, then I wanted to go ahead and just get the surgery done and be done with everything."

Becoming ready for the BRCA test and all its emotional, medical, and personal consequences is an intensely personal experience. It's impossible to determine exactly what factors will allow a woman to realize she's ready to start the next chapter in her life, beginning with testing. As one woman put it, "Everything started falling into place." A woman is ready to get tested when she finally wants to know: am I BRCA positive?

BRCA Testing: A Family Affair

As we have seen, one of a woman's biggest considerations in deciding on the BRCA test is her family. Every woman I interviewed discussed how her family influenced her decision in some way. For example, Sam described how her mother, grandfather, and two aunts were diagnosed with cancer before Sam herself was tested.

The mutation obviously came from my grandpa who had already passed away from pancreatic cancer. So, at that time I wasn't old enough to test, and I had to wait until I must have been maybe fourteen? Fifteen? So younger, too young for it. And I always knew that I would have the test done. So when I was eighteen-years-old, the children's hospital contacted me because they had done it all on a research basis. No one had to pay for it, um, so they contacted me when I turned eighteen, and I said, "Yeah, I would love to have the test done." I went in, had it done, and I knew before I got there that I was gonna be positive. It was just an assumption. Um, I was gonna be positive. Yeah, I mean, growing up I thought that I was going to have cancer. It was always, from the time I was little, I was always going to have cancer. It was always talked about. Everyone always had cancer. You know, it was everywhere.

Many women seek out the BRCA test because of a strong family history of breast or ovarian cancer. Or a sudden diagnosis or death in the family can be the final spark that sends a woman to the doctor's office. Family history can either motivate a woman to do some research and find out about the BRCA mutation or indicate to her doctor that BRCA testing is the right step. Some women get tested after another close family member tests positive, whether following a recent cancer diagnosis or not. Of the women I interviewed, 83 percent had another BRCA-positive relative and 81 percent had a relative who had been diagnosed with cancer. One woman's positive result or cancer diagnosis can often spur a chain reaction of testing among family members.

Susan's mother was diagnosed with breast cancer ten years before our interview. At the time, her family didn't think it was a big deal because the cancer wasn't that aggressive. Eight years later, though, Susan's oldest sister (in her thirties) was diagnosed with breast cancer. The genetic connection was too obvious to ignore. Her two older sisters were tested immediately, and after doing some more research Susan got tested as well.

I went to a young survivor's coalition conference with my sister and my mother and my other sister. . . . And so it was all pre-menopausal women, so a lot of young women with cancer. And, you know, and I started going to these breakout groups where they would talk about all the side effects of chemotherapy and . . . that conference really, like, jarred, that really jarred me. I felt like, I actually felt scared of the chemotherapy. I was like, I wasn't so scared of the breast cancer for some reason, I was really scared of, like, losing my hair and then potentially losing my fertility if I got chemotherapy and, um, I don't know. It just, it was just, I didn't want to be single and have chemotherapy [laughs] and, like, lose my looks as well, you know? So—And that is like, a light bulb went off. All of a sudden, I was like, wait, why can't I get a mastectomy? I remember the moment it happened, I was on a bus and I just all of a sudden was like, I think I could do it. Like, if it could save me from cancer and chemo, then maybe this isn't so out of this, you know, out of the realm of reality. So, that's when I got tested.

Watching loved ones struggle with cancer diagnoses, chemotherapy, and often death can leave no question in a woman's mind that BRCA testing will help them. If they can find out their risk, how could they not do something about it? One woman described her mother as "the martyr and pioneer, dying . . . so that all of us [in the family] could get tested for the gene to get our boobs cut off" and to prevent cancer. Another woman got tested without hesitation as soon as her doctor suggested it because she had seen her mother die of breast cancer and had a daughter of her own. Getting tested enabled her to have preventive surgery and "beat cancer."

BRCA testing ends the cycle of cancer and death that plagues many families. Stephanie is one woman who wanted to get tested as soon as she found out it was an option. She is in her thirties and married with two children that she cares for full time. To her, testing was a no-brainer: her maternal grandmother, two aunts, and mother had all been diagnosed with breast cancer. "When I was eighteen, I remember hearing about the gene mutation testing they were doing and thinking to myself, 'Well of course, I'm going to do that.' . . . So, actually, as a young adult I knew I would take the test." Because all the women in her family had been diagnosed, she always wondered "not if, but when" she would be diagnosed as well. For much of her life, Stephanie was waiting for cancer to come.

Once her two daughters were born and Stephanie was about thirty years old, she decided it was time to get tested. She wanted to get preventive surgery so she could be around for her children and avoid the fate of her mother, who just had her third reoccurrence of breast cancer. Her mother was the first in the family to be tested and having that history of positive results in the family ensured that Stephanie's insurance would cover her own test. BRCA testing allowed her to start "the next phase of [her] life."

I felt like I had this weight on my shoulders this whole life wondering when cancer was going to strike me. And I just was having that strong pull to kind of deal with this, be done with it for the most part, and then just start, you know, the next phase of my life, you know, with kind of a new outlook on my future. And you know, I have two young girls at home, and I just, to me it was something that I needed to do and needed to do quickly. I wasn't pressed by any doctors or anything to do it quickly. There was no, you know, no cancer scare. My path reports came back clean, nothing like precancer or anything. That was just my own personal drive to not just sit on the information. After I educated myself, you know, I learned all that I could learn. I made up my mind pretty quickly on how I wanted to go about it as far as what type of reconstruction and stuff like that. So I just was like, "Let's do it." . . . I pretty much was convinced that it was going to be not a matter of if, but when.

Women like Stephanie's mother provide the spark for a testing chain reaction in their families. They're the informants: they share what they've learned about the BRCA mutation and the benefits of being tested. One woman noted, "My dad was pushing me into looking into getting tested." Sisters, aunts, and mothers will tell their family about the test and encourage them to take it. Some women will take on a proactive role by collecting hereditary information about the BRCA mutation and cancer diagnoses and tracing their family's BRCA history back in time. Women play the role of informant when they feel it is their moral obligation or "genetic responsibility" to tell family members about the risk (Kenen 1994; Novas and Rose 2000, 5).

In Lauren's family, her aunt was the informant. Her aunt developed breast cancer and underwent chemotherapy as well as breast surgery, and over time became the proactive member of her family in dealing with their risk of cancer. As Lauren described:

She does a lot of research about our family history. She's kind of like the Hallmark person in our family who's like, "Oh, have you heard about this new thing? Or this new diet?" Or, you know, "Make sure you're eating well," or, "I'm gonna do this alternative cancer practice." And, and so I've been influenced by her.

Lauren notes that it was easier to know she might carry the BRCA mutation because of her aunt's support throughout her teenage years. Relying on her aunt's support and knowledge allowed Lauren to gradually make lifestyle changes that would improve her chances of not getting cancer and, ultimately, to get tested.

BRCA testing really becomes a family affair when women get tested together, as a way to support one another. One woman who got tested with her older sister told me, "We're both in it together." Lauren has a strong history of the BRCA mutation in her family and she's known about the presence of the BRCA gene in her family since she was fifteen. Lauren notes, "I think, [getting tested] was definitely triggered, [by my mom] 'cause she was sort of looking out for us and was concerned and was curious to know if we had the gene or not. . . . She left it up to us, but we decided to do it and get tested at the same time so that we would find out . . . together." When Lauren was nineteen, she and her sister were tested and both were positive. As she recalls it, finding out her BRCA-positive status felt like a confirmation of what she already knew: "I had known about the presence of the gene for so long that getting tested was kind of, like, just an affirmation, because it was maybe four years earlier when I was fifteen when I first became conscious that there was this gene that ran in my family that I had a 50 chance of having."

Their family's past alone doesn't motivate women to get tested, but also future generations. Women get tested for themselves and for the sake of close family members who also may be at risk. Sisters want to inspire each other to take control of their health. Mothers want a fighting chance to survive cancer and be around for their children. Any woman can pass critical information about the BRCA mutation on to her children and other relatives to encourage them to also get tested. Older women are especially motivated to take advantage of the new opportunities of medical technology that will allow younger generations to be proactive in the fight against cancer. Some women get tested almost entirely for selfless reasons. I spoke with one woman who actually didn't want to get tested but did anyway for her sister: "How could I do that to my sister, how could I prevent her from knowing?"

When it comes to family, though, children come to the fore. Women want to save their children from losing their mother and give them knowledge about their own cancer risk. One-third of the women I interviewed were married and over half had at least one child. As we saw, Stephanie was motivated to get tested for the BRCA mutation based on her family's history of breast cancer, but her children were the final and crucial factor.

I didn't want my kids in the future to watch me go through cancer and chemo like I had with my mom. So actually, as a young adult, I knew I would take the test . . . And then after I gave birth to both my girls, I figured it was a good time to go ahead and address the issue. So I took the test. . . . And then later on that year I had the prophylactic mastectomy because I was about to turn thirty. I was twenty-nine, and I had it in my head that I really wanted to start the next decade of my life, you know, with better odds against cancer and without worry, so that was my plan.

The "biggest" factor that made her ready to get tested was being married, having kids, and wanting to be able to "stay around longer" for them.

Stephanie's two daughters are both still young, but she is already reflecting on the future of BRCA in their lives—she thinks about it "more than you can even imagine." Although she feels guilty knowing that she may have passed on the BRCA mutation, she hopes she has also set a "good example" for them, so they will be proactive about their own health. All told, the thoughts of past and future generations weigh heavily on women as they make important decisions about BRCA testing.

Not Ready for Cancer to Come

Well, it sort of began when I was fifteen, when my mother was tested. She had already survived breast cancer, and she was part of one of the first studies done in California, and so, they wanted to test me, and at the time, there wasn't any, um, I believe that laws weren't in place for health care companies to, you know, protect people that had genetic illnesses. So I, along with my parents, we decided that that just wasn't a good idea to get me tested because I might have been dropped from my health care. And also, I don't really think—they didn't really offer preventative surgeries for anyone that was fifteen. What they wanted to do, if I had tested positive, they wanted to have me take this drug that would have dissolved all of the fat in my breasts and [laughing], and I just wasn't prepared to do that at fifteen. It just seemed . . . and so, this whole time, it's been in the back of my mind.

Being ready for the BRCA test doesn't always happen as soon as women—or girls like Jenna—learn about the option. Many hold off for years or even decades before getting tested. Some aren't ready to be tested even though they feel they already knew they were BRCA positive. Most of the women who wait so long seem no different from those who do not—they have a strong history of breast and ovarian cancer and even the BRCA mutation in their families. So why don't they rush to get tested? We've already seen the answer: becoming ready can be a process that happens over time. Jenna is one woman who waited to get tested until, as she described it, the "perfect storm" of factors fell into place.

Jenna was in her early thirties when I interviewed her. As we saw, Jenna was only a teenager when she learned her mother was BRCA positive. Her mother had been diagnosed with breast cancer and entered a clinical study that included genetic testing. Unfortunately, Jenna's mother's battle with the BRCA mutation was not over. She had a second recurrence of breast cancer when Jenna was in her early twenties, four years later was also diagnosed with ovarian cancer, and died shortly thereafter.

Jenna spoke with me about growing up in the shadow of her mother's cancer diagnosis and constantly trying to save the memories that they knew would be cut short: "Intellectually I felt like she was maybe going to be okay, but emotionally I like held on to everything because I sort of knew my time with her was going to be like super short." Jenna always felt, though, that because she wasn't sick like her mom, she shouldn't worry about getting cancer.

> My mom's survival totally trumped, like, any worries that I had about myself. Totally, because I wasn't sick, you know, she was the one that was actually going through it. You know, it was just like, the problem was like intellectual exercise as opposed to, like, well if there was real shit going on, I gotta, you know, keep my eye on the ball with my mom.

Once her mother passed away, though, she felt a sense of survivor's guilt, a guilt that recently reemerged with a cousin's cancer diagnosis and radiation treatment (Douglas, Hamilton, and Grubs 2009).

Jenna's risk perception changed over time. As a teenager, she was so concerned about her mother's cancer and the threat that it would reoccur that she didn't reflect on her own risk. In her twenties, she was focused on her mother's second recurrence of breast cancer—which had progressed to stage IV—as well her mother's development of ovarian cancer and eventual death. It was only in her later twenties that Jenna began to focus on her own risk of getting cancer and, based on her mother's timeline, she gave herself a death sentence.

Such fatalism at first kept her from BRCA testing because, in her mind, it would only confirm her worst fears. Getting cancer and being BRCA positive became for Jenna, and for many of the women I spoke with, one and the same—an idea we discuss further in chapter 4. She told me, "I also was really, really scared. I think, in fact, I was really just chicken, to get the test done. It was sort of like an ostrich, like I'm just going to pretend, you know, if I don't think about it, then I'm not going to have to worry about it." Jenna also didn't feel rushed to get the test at such a young age. She was able to place cancer "at bay." By choosing not to be tested, she could actually open up some space in her life to normalize her situation and to gain some control over her cancer risk.

It was in her early thirties that a "perfect storm" came together that made her rethink the decision not to get tested. Her cousin's more recent cancer diagnosis, along with Jenna's own cancer scare and her supportive husband, were all factors that drove her to get tested.

> And, you know, it was right before I got married. I'd been with my husband, you know, we've been together for six years, but. . . . We were, you know, planning on, on getting married, and it just seemed like, okay I'm thirty-four, like I'm not . . . I gotta face up to the music; I'm not in my twenties. . . . And so, there was sort of like, you know, a perfect storm, like everything sort of fell into place. And I just realized that I gotta get this done, I gotta find out if I have this gene, and if I do, you know, I can't really fool around. . . . So I got it done, and then two weeks later I found out that I am BRCA positive.

For Jenna and for many other women, deciding to get the BRCA test is neither a simple nor an immediate decision. It's also not an empowering one in and of itself, despite the way Myriad Corporation frames it, as we saw in chapter 1. Just checking off a prompt about family history on the Be Ready Quiz from Myriad's BRACAnalysis® website would not accurately inform Jenna's testing decision. In fact, one woman might check yes to all the questions on this quiz and still not be personally ready for the test. A woman's decision to get tested is an ongoing, time-consuming, and complex process that involves her family, friends, "sisters," and much more.

As Jenna showed me, delaying the test can be a helpful strategy to "buy time" and create a sense of normalcy in women's lives. A woman can accomplish important life goals before she formally confirms her BRCA-positive status and addresses her cancer risk. Before devoting the time and energy to their fight against cancer, many women want to live without that fear and reach life goals such as finishing their education, launching a career, finding a partner, and having children. Delaying the test is not the same as ignoring a high cancer risk. Some women do all of the things a medical doctor might tell any young high-risk woman to do—such as eating healthily and practicing a higher surveillance routine with more frequent mammograms and check-ups—but they delay the final confirmation that they are BRCA positive. Carving out this liminal space allows women to gain some power and control over their cancer risk.

Who Gets Tested . . . And Who Doesn't Even Get the Chance?

It is important to point out that some women's voices are missing from this book altogether: women who never even consider or never get the opportunity to get tested for the BRCA mutation. So who are the women who are forgotten by the world of genetic testing? Let's look first at who does. Of the women I interviewed, 90 percent were Caucasian, 80 percent identified themselves as middle class, and none said they were lower class. They were well educated, too: 90 percent had at least an associate's degree. So my own small study suggests that women who get tested are very alike: white, middle class, and well educated.

It would seem that systemic racial, cultural, and socioeconomic barriers—such as a lack of financial resources and misinformation about BRCA testing—keep women who are not white, well educated, and well-off from being tested. These same factors could have also affected my ability to recruit diverse women to my study. In other words, unequal access to BRCA testing reflects the disparity that is endemic to our health-care system and that prevents many women from making comprehensive and informed decisions about their health.

How a woman learns about BRCA testing often influences her understanding of her true cancer risk, as well as of the proper steps she should take. Some learn about the BRCA mutation from advertising by genetic testing agencies. Dana, whom we met in chapter 1, found out this way. Her aunt contacted her with informational material from Myriad Laboratory. So much information and responsibility in the hands of one company opens up the possibility that women will receive incorrect or incomplete information. Furthermore, some companies disperse testing information to targeted areas of the country, which leaves decisions about who learns about BRCA testing up to the whim (and financial interests) of private corporations. Although these firms provide useful information, in the end they are for-profit industries that thrive on more women getting tested, not necessarily on women's well-being. Women can also be at the mercy of their health-care providers and the limited number of genetic counselors available to provide accurate and comprehensive information about the test, its cost, and its possible repercussions (Tambor, Rimer, and Strigo 1997, 44). Poor women are the most likely to be affected by geographical barriers, low-quality health care, and a lack of access to specialists such as oncologists and genetic counselors.

Race is also a barrier to access. White women are disproportionably tested for hereditary breast cancer. In the doctor's chair, they are more often presented with the possibility of being BRCA positive and with their options for testing (Hall et al. 2009). Women of color, especially women of African ethnicity, are tested very little despite actually having a high rate of the BRCA mutation (Hall et al. 2009). Because the majority of medical studies on hereditary breast cancer are done in white communities, women of color may often have a poor understanding or opinion of genetic testing (Lagos et al. 2008). As we know that greater awareness of BRCA correlates strongly with the desire to be tested, lack of knowledge of the gene in nonwhite communities is an important barrier to getting tested (Mogilner et al. 1998). This fact is disturbing in light of the racial diversity that genetic testing agencies, and Myriad in particular, show in their advertisements. Why show such diversity when, in fact, the population of women getting tested is much more homogeneous?

Various cultural traditions and beliefs can also factor into women's decision-making. People in the Latina community, for example, traditionally experience lower levels of social support for genetic testing (Lagos et al. 2008). This circumstance creates a barrier to testing for many Latin women; as we have seen, with weak social support networks, women are less likely to follow cancer preventive guidelines and pursue the option of genetic testing. In addition, a Chinese woman I interviewed was conflicted between her decision to get tested and her family's cultural beliefs. According to June, her family and others in the Chinese community think testing is silly and didn't support her decision to be tested at all. We discuss June's experiences further in chapters 3, 4, and 7.

The amount that BRCA testing is marketed to white women has led to a disturbing trend: many of the women getting tested don't actually have a high risk for the BRCA mutation. Instead of being driven by personal or family experience, women are being driven by advertisements. Studies have shown that risk perception is a greater motivator for testing than actual risk, and, with increases in the marketing and accessibility of genetic testing, more and more women are being tested—many more than need to be (Pilarski 2009). When testing companies oversimplify risk factors, they drive many women to spend time and money on testing they do not need. Although the BRCA mutation accounts for only a tiny fraction of the 5–10 percent of hereditary breast cancer cases, when many women view Myriad's direct-to-consumer (DTC) advertisements, they "self-refer" themselves to their family physicians (White et al. 2008, 2980). The number of women using genetic services increased 240 percent after Myriad's DTC marketing campaign for BRCAnalysis®. This spike in demand delayed access to counseling and testing for those who truly needed it (White et al. 2008)·

The results of other studies confirm that the women I spoke with are fairly representative of all women who are tested in the United States: white, middle- to upper-class women who have the education to learn of the test and the insurance or money to pay for it. Their cultural background does not bar genetic testing as a viable option to fight cancer. Most of the literature about BRCA testing and genetic testing in general actually remains limited to these demographics. While this book tells the stories of some women of color and others from underserved communities, we often don't hear these underrepresented voices.

Here's what we have heard: women follow a lot of different paths on their route to BRCA testing. Being told they are BRCA positive may be a relief for some women—they finally know the truth. But for others it may be an unexpected shock. Although they have taken the first steps in their journey, they're still waiting for cancer to come. BRCA-positive mutation women have many steps to take, including assessing their cancer risk and making decisions about prevention. The next chapter explores how women receive and share the news that they are BRCA positive. We'll start to see how women look to the future while they are waiting for cancer to come.

THREE

"You're BRCA Positive"

Those aren't easy words to hear. But at age twenty-eight, Christina describes how disempowering it can feel to spend her whole life waiting for cancer to come.

My mom was diagnosed with breast cancer at age thirty. You know, I'm not that far away from that age. I'm twenty-nine this fall and thirty is going to be soon after. And I think that, you know, just the impact of having a sick mother when you're little, you know, I've been afraid of cancer my whole life. My whole life I've been feeling like I have to attain to my mother's sort of life schedule. I think she also got married at twenty-seven or whatever.

You know, when I was young I used to say I'm going to be married by like twenty-four, and I want to go ahead and have my kids at like twenty-seven or whatever so that when I get cancer, not if I get cancer, but when I get breast cancer at a stupidly young age, I've already accomplished some of these life milestones. So, you know, my life is not following my mother's plan now. But, um, there was a very real sense of, "I'm getting close to my mother's diagnosis date and do I, you know, do I want to try to play chicken with my life?"

I actually had the misfortune that when I recently got my genetic news, a week later, my grandfather died, my dad's father died, and then a week after that my mother's mother died. So, um, I was carrying around my testing news to all these funerals. My aunt and I went by to give my grandmother's things to a breast cancer house that offers such things to low-income women. And my, my aunt kept saying to me, "It's okay to feel crazy." I was a wreck.

Later, in the weeks and months leading up to my mastectomy,

we were just talking about it a little bit for the first time, and she was saying that she always felt growing up that if she could just make it to thirty without cancer then she knew she would be okay. And she said, "And I made it to thirty, and then I thought, if I could just make it to thirty-five without getting cancer, then I would be, you know, then I know I would be okay. Then I would be happy." And she said, you know, she made it to thirty-five, and she was just tired of waiting at that point. And that coupled with my mother urging, um, my aunt to do this. Um, those two things combined, um, led my aunt to, uh, go ahead and get the mastectomy.

Christina has a strong family history of cancer, but it took her years to be ready to hear the words "you're BRCA positive." Her mother was diagnosed at age thirty, so Christina always assumed she'd also be BRCA positive and get cancer. She even thought she'd follow her mother's exact timeline. Still, when she finally got the positive result, she was upset, felt unprepared, and went on antidepressants: "When I got that genetic news it was just like every day was full of pain and terror." These emotions are common for women facing hereditary breast cancer and dealing with the confusing guidance that often comes with a BRCA-positive result. Christina doesn't know what to believe.

With a BRCA-positive result comes important medical decisions. But, before women make choices about prevention, they often have a lot of work to do to learn what their results mean for them and for their families. Some women come from family backgrounds riddled with cancer and feel more prepared for the fight. These women may have been exploring their options for years. Other women are shocked by the positive BRCA result. In a few months, they have to make the decisions that others have had so long to consider.

Deciding whether or how to tell her family about her test results is a complex process that's different for every woman (Wilson and Etchegary 2010). Her family's reaction will change how she takes in the information. Some women are empowered by their families' love and support. Others are disempowered when their families don't want to be told about the BRCA results. Some families are completely unsupportive of a woman's decision to get tested or get preventive surgery in order to fight cancer before it develops.

In this chapter, as we weave in and out of women's stories about learning they are BRCA-positive mutation carriers and sharing this news with their loved ones, we consider many questions. How to women react to learning they are BRCA positive? How does the support or rejection of family members affect how they understand and use this information? Do women reach out to their families to inform them of their own possible genetic risks? Most important, how can the experiences of these women help others in the future?

Getting the News

Some women are relieved when they find out they're BRCA positive. They feel liberated and armed with the knowledge they need to fight cancer. The positive result is a confirmation of what they already knew if they come from families with a strong history of cancer. Now they can get on with their lives and make plans to do whatever they need to do to "beat the cancer clock." Some even feel lucky because genetic testing wasn't an option for their beloved family members who have struggled with cancer.

Others feel caught off guard by the news. They feel shock and disbelief. Even when these women know that cancer runs in the family, even when they have watched a close family member die of cancer, they may have never actually linked this medical history to the possibility of a hereditary gene. For these women, a medical professional first mentions BRCA. Getting the test can be extremely disempowering when women are suddenly faced with the fear and the decisions that BRCA positivity entails. But however the women in my study respond, by noting that getting the positive results overwhelming increases the importance of BRCA in their lives such that they feel that "BRCA and all it involves" takes up 22 percent of their lives six months before the BRCA test, but that sentiment rises to 66 percent of their lives six months after the test.

Let's look at Stephanie and Marla's stories about discovering their BRCA status and sharing that news with their families. Reading them side by side will help us unpack the complexity of this journey. One narrative is more upbeat in tone than the other, but both show that every woman experiences a uniquely personal blend of confidence and insecurity, of affirmation and denial, when she faces her BRCA positivity.

"I Already Knew": Stephanie's Story

To recap, Stephanie, whom we first met in chapter 2, is thirty-one and a married, stay-at-home mom with two children. She has a strong history of breast cancer in her family: her mother has had breast cancer three times and is currently fighting a metastatic, stage IV recurrence. Most cancer survivors in her family were diagnosed in their forties and fifties, so she wants to have an oophorectomy in her thirties. She already had a mastectomy. This way, she feels she can start fresh in this decade, without BRCA to worry about.

Stephanie was calm when she first got the BRCA news. Because of her family history, she wasn't surprised: "It was like I already knew."

> I've never freaked out about it. I've never, I've never taken it as like a really horrible thing. I don't know, I just kind of have the personality that, "Hey, whatever, it is what it is. Let's just roll with it." I just kind of feel like I've been prepped my whole life for dealing with this. . . . It wasn't even like that big of a deal if that makes sense. I mean, yes, it crushed me. When I found out the results, even though I knew she was going to say yes, I still sat there and cried like an idiot, you know. But it just—yeah. It was just something that I kind of always knew and dealt with.

Many women feel that testing positive for the BRCA mutation is inevitable. Learning the results brings a sense of empowerment—finally they can take action, usually preventive surgery, to eradicate their cancer risk.

Stephanie's family situation made it a quick decision to have preventive bilateral mastectomy. She is planning to have her ovaries removed by her thirty-fifth birthday: a fairly easy decision because she is married and doesn't plan to have more children. She also wants the surgery for the sake of her children, so she will be around long enough to see them grow up.

Stephanie also found comfort in her marriage and faith. She has the support of her husband, without whom her experience would be much more difficult. And they are comfortable enough financially to pay for testing and preventive measures. She had good insurance coverage, unlike many others. Her faith also provided support. "I believe in God," she notes. "I believe that my whole life I've just been prepped for certain things . . . given the personality that I have because God must have known that I'd be facing this type of stuff eventually." After completing her preventive surgery, Stephanie had a cross tattooed on her ankle. What does that signify? "God had my back," she explains.

All of these factors play a role in Stephanie's feeling empowered by the test and by taking action to turn around her genetic destiny. Her story mirrors what the genetic testing industry advertises to women: knowledge is power.

As Stephanie says, "I wanted to start the next decade of my life with better odds against cancer." And knowing she is BRCA positive provided a "strong pull to kind of deal with this, be done with it." As Stephanie explains, "I feel like I'm facing a clean slate, a new start," a future that will now be open for good things, "whereas before there was a dark cloud."

Caught Off Guard: Marla's Story

For some women, getting the news that they're BRCA positive is a shock they're not ready to face. Some women are advised by a health-care provider to get tested because they've experienced a cancer scare or diagnosis. They might not have done much research or didn't really think they'd be positive. For some, unsettled personal circumstances make this news too much to bear.

Marla is a university administrator in her early forties. She got divorced in her thirties and has two children. With an African-American mother and Italian father, she identifies herself as biracial. Marla knows there is a strong history of breast and ovarian cancer on both sides of her family. She lost her mother to ovarian cancer and her aunt on her father's side to breast cancer. But cancer was not something the family ever talked about when Marla was growing up. And family members did not want the BRCA test. As Marla puts it:

> I had an aunt that died of breast cancer; it wasn't really something that was talked about in my family. She died before I was born. I never thought about breast cancer. So . . . discovering my lump myself in the shower at the age of thirty-six, it didn't occur to me that it could have been breast cancer. It really didn't dawn on me, um, you know, kind of strange, but I did decide to go to the doctor because it was, you know, not normal. But I never thought about breast cancer until I laid down on the doctor's bed, and he had that look in his face, and I thought, "Uh oh."

Taking her family's cancer history into consideration, Marla's surgeon suggested that she be tested for the BRCA mutation. Marla was "anxious and nervous throughout the whole testing process." But she never hesitated when it came to being tested: "I really didn't, no there wasn't a question in my mind about whether I would have the test. I have a daughter and a son, so I wanted to make sure we were informed." Marla then used what she learned to decide whether she should have one or both of her breasts removed. "I decided to have both my breasts removed because of the result of the genetic test. So my doctor had me do testing before the surgery so we could make a decision about whether or not I'd have a bilateral mastectomy."

Marla's extended family members knew about her cancer diagnosis and testing, but didn't get the test themselves. Marla explains:

> My family knew that I was having the test, and I anticipated that they would, as well, have the test. I thought it would be an automatic kind of thing, as a result of what I was going through. They chose not to. They all, you know, individually, made decisions and felt as though they didn't want that information. I think they just felt like, you know, if they were going to get breast cancer, they'd get it. And if they didn't they don't. And they didn't want something sort of hanging over their head saying it was coming, I guess. They preferred to just go on with their lives without getting tested.

Marla's testing experience had elements of both empowerment and disempowerment. Marla gained some agency when learning the news thanks to the support of her genetics counselor and doctors.

> The counselors were wonderful. They explained the procedure, they explained some of the research around genetic testing, and it just was very, very comfortable. I then felt comfortable about going through with the testing at that time . . . I relied on my doctors. I had one of the best surgeons in the country, and I knew that I was in good hands. I trusted that, and I know not everyone can. I felt connected with my doctor.

Marla felt comfortable with her decisions about being testing and about having preventive surgery. She provided her family, especially her children, with important information about their potential risk for hereditary cancer.

On the other hand, Marla's decision to proceed with testing, unlike that of many women who undergo testing, was not approved and supported by her extended family. Instead, it estranged her from her family. And now she feels disempowered to do anything about those severed relationships.

> I think they were maybe just in denial and didn't want anything to confirm that they might also be at risk. I never really had a discussion

with my family in terms of really working that whole thing out. In fact, they weren't very supportive throughout my process. . . . Once we got through those initial stages of discovering the breast cancer, and some of those other initial stages. They weren't supportive. . . . In fact, it's had a significant negative impact on the way I relate to my family, something I've struggled with since then. Um, because you know, I expected that they would be my rock, my support. And that wasn't the case at all.

Marla's children were also devastated by the news of her BRCA-positive status. Deciding to remove her breasts and ovaries had both ill and positive effects on her family relationships.

My kids were devastated. My son was away at boarding school at the time, and he tried to get kicked out. He did some things—he knew that I wanted him to stay, but he really felt that he wanted to be home taking care of me. My daughter has an underlying fear that she's going to get cancer when she's my age. She had a really difficult time with the news. She stopped eating for a while and lost a lot of weight. I think, on the other hand, this experience ultimately made us a stronger family as well.

Luckily, Marla's friends were there for her when her family was not: "I was fighting for my life every day. While I had the support of friends, I ultimately did not have my family's support."

Marla and Stephanie were making BRCA decisions in very different contexts. Marla was at a later stage of life and was living with only her youngest child at home. She had no husband and no extended family for support. Stephanie had the benefit of many years to get herself ready to make these decisions. In the meantime, she was able to create the life that she had envisioned for herself. Marla is just beginning to come to terms with her BRCA status and the surgical decision she quickly made. She was forced into testing because of her cancer diagnosis, but she also wanted to gather information for her children's sake. Although seven years have passed since she made those decisions, Marla still feels her life is "a work in progress."

Deciding Who to Tell

After getting their results, one of the biggest decisions women have to make is how, when, and if to tell their family. For some women, it's an easy decision. After all, they got tested for the sake of others who might also be at risk—their children, siblings, and extended family members. So telling their blood relatives about their BRCA risk feels like a moral obligation. Yet some women worry about this decision. Exactly whom should they tell? Should they consider a relative's potential risk? What about age? The decision is even more complicated when some relatives are out of the communication loop or on bad terms. Deciding just whom to tell your news, how to tell them, and when to tell them requires careful thought. Most women do share the news with someone, more often than not a close first-degree relative. Researchers say that over 90 percent of women will share the news with at least one other person (Julian-Reynier 2000). Deciding to share the news will depend on the woman's age; whether she has daughters; the woman's own familial cancer history; whether she is single, married, or divorced; and the extent of her emotional involvement with family members.

Women often get tested for the sake of their children, but then feel guilty about passing on their "bad genes" and worry about what will happen if their children are positive. Because of this guilt, women will sometimes withhold genetic information from their children. They want to ignore the possibility that they have given their children anything but the best of themselves. Parents especially avoid telling very young children, whom they believe cannot fully understand or handle the news.

But most mothers do tell their children about the BRCA mutation. Those who do are influenced by the age of their child, his or her relative maturity, and the immediate relevance of the information to their child's life (Forrest et al. 2003; Huff 2010; Peshkin, DeMarco, and Tercyak 2010). It's a difficult decision. The longer a woman waits to disclose the information to her children, the longer she puts them at risk. But risk-reduction surgery and other preventive options are generally not recommended until age twenty-five, so sharing this news with young children has little or no medical benefit (MacKenzie, Patrick-Miller, and Bradbury 2009). The benefits are still there. Older children can often be a source of support for mothers who learn they're BRCA positive. Andrea, who received no support from her husband, found it instead in her eighteen-year-old daughter. Andrea explains, "She loves to go on the breast cancer walk with me and she feels real proud we're surviving families, you know, that I survived it."

In some cases, the results are kept a secret from some close family members but not others. Marion's mother and sister kept the results from her for some time. She was only in her twenties when her mother was diagnosed with breast cancer. So Marion knew about testing, but she "didn't want to know" her status, even though, as she explains, "I felt like I would be a ticking time bomb, kind of waiting for it" to be positive. She was too young for the test, she decided, and would have no idea what to do with the information except to wait for cancer to come. Years later, her sister was also diagnosed with cancer and wanted the test. Marion's mother got tested first, although she and Marion's sister kept the results from Marion for some time. Marion is "very sensitive," they explained. In fact, when Marion was in college, she wasn't even told that her mother had breast surgery.

Looking back, Marion is now glad she has the information. It's encouraged her to learn about preventive surgery and to have a mastectomy. In the end, Marion's family revealed what had been kept from her and helped her decide to be tested. But the secrets that relatives keep can be extremely stressful on later relationships—and even on their very health. Claire's family provides a striking example.

Claire's Story: Keeping Family Secrets

I guarantee you, what I'm about to say will shock you. Okay? So my older sister, to my knowledge, she was the first to find out. And I think my mother told my sister, uh, right around the time when she was tested. Because I think in families when you have three siblings, there's always going to be the pecking order. I've always been in the middle. I'm sometimes the first to know, I'm sometimes the last to know. And my not knowing, my finding out that I was not "in the know," if you will, did not surprise me. Because as the middle child, I think my mother felt—she went to have all this testing done, and I'm not sure if my mother was listening closely to the geneticist, but I don't believe my mother when she says that she was told not to tell all three children at one time. I don't believe that my being a new mother meant that I couldn't handle this, whatever the outcome.

I think that this has changed my relationship with both of my parents in a big way. Because I don't know when exactly they were going to tell me. I had to find out for myself through my—through my obstetrician who urged me to find out more about my mother's hysterectomy. So there's a lot of, um, I'm sort of suspicious about, about this information because I feel like it was withheld from me. And my older sister already knew this information. It was withheld from me for three months. Three months! And in my mother's mind, "What's three months? It's not a big deal. I was going to tell you. There's no cancer in my family." You know, on and on and on and on. She was making excuses that I don't agree with. And as a family, I think that we're old enough and mature enough to sit down together and have an open discussion about it . . .

I don't like secrets, but I feel like it was information that I needed to have. And on that note, I want to say that my younger sister knows nothing about the fact that my mother tested positive for the BRCA mutation. She is totally in the dark. My mother has made excuse after excuse after excuse, based on her own situation and some of the struggling she's been through with other family members. There have been a lot of things that have been going on in my mother's life. So she feels that when the time is right she will tell my younger sister. And at that time they will then, you know, do what I did, which was, you know, start the process.

And my sister may be negative. And I think, my older sister testing negative, it made my mother think, "What's the likelihood of me being positive? [My oldest daughter] was negative." But in my genetic counseling session, the geneticist made it very clear to me, in front of my mother, that every sibling is different. You can even have one sibling that is positive and two that are negative. My younger sister doesn't know anything about the real reason for my mother's hysterectomy and that I am positive for the BRCA mutation as well as my mom. She knows nothing about any of this.

My parents and I have been back and forth about this. It has sort of been made very clear to me that this is none of my business anymore, that they are going to deal with my younger sister on their terms and on their own timeline. Because they feel that, um, maybe—just getting back to the family dynamics here, I think they feel that as the youngest of three girls, there is an even more protective nature—I don't know how to put this—but they're more protective of her because she's younger, and they feel she's more immature and won't take the information in quite the same way that I did, like an adult, like a mature adult.

They may be surprised by her response. But at the same time, that's been an issue for me. So all of this knowledge has changed how I see my parents in a big way, and in a short period of time, because the two of them, I don't think, understand that although my mother didn't have cancer or my sister didn't have cancer, that having the BRCA mutation is like a family history.

They are keeping secrets that are health-related. Of all secrets to be keeping—and that's why I went immediately to my psychotherapist, who I trust and love. I wanted her to honestly tell me how she feels about this. And she said, "This is not good." [laughing] Because she said, "It's so interesting what your parents choose to . . ." Um, we're such an enmeshed family, but yet over issues so vital, vital health issues, um, they have taken a whole other position . . .

I think I do share a little bit of my parents' concern. But I also think that she is thirty years old, and this perhaps may open up her world to, um, being an adult. I don't know how to put it. This is, this is what real adults deal with. And in the end, she could be negative. So all this worry is for nothing. And as my therapist said to me, "Every month that your mother waits is . . ." I don't know exactly, what her exact words were, but she was saying, "It's not good to wait." I want you to know, I have in, um, a very light-hearted, casual way, I said to my mother, "I have concerns about your not telling her this information yet."

I am now part of the secret keeping. Which is very hard for me. Because of the two—of all three girls, I am the one who comes clean the fastest, who has the guilty conscience. . . . Who feels like . . . I really want to please my parents. I'm married and I have a son, but I still want to do right by my mother and father, because I appreciate everything that they have done for me. My older sister wants to please my parents in a different way. She's like a team player as far as the secret keeping, but I'm not. I don't agree with it.

You know, I haven't talked with my parents about my younger sister in the last few weeks. It hasn't come up. But I wanted, for my own piece of mind, to let my mother know that I have serious concerns about her withholding this information given what I just went through. When the radiologist said, and my mother was in the room with me, "Your MRI is scary, Claire." I looked at her. I looked at her and I said, "Mom, what do you think?" And she just, her eyes popped, and she said, "I cannot believe this." And I didn't—I don't think I cried once throughout this process. Because I knew at the bottom of my heart, or my soul, that anything that this was early was salvageable. So I had the confidence in the doctor, um, I was actually more concerned about my younger sister, crazy as that may sound [laughing].

Claire's mother originally hid from her the presence of the BRCA mutation in the family, only telling her oldest sister and keeping this information from Claire and her younger sister. Claire guesses that her mother "needed a little more time." Even when Claire learned about her family's BRCA-positive mutation history, her mother pressured her and her older sister to keep the information from her younger sister. Claire has complied, but she has reservations. Deciding whom to tell isn't easy. Claire's story makes that clear. There are many family members that become involved, relationships to maintain, personalities to deal with, and the fear of cancer looming over everything. Most families don't resort to keeping secrets from close relatives, but all struggle with these same issues.

Sharing the News

Revealing her BRCA-positive status can be good or bad for a woman and her family. Whatever the consequences, many women feel not only a responsibility but also a moral obligation to share their BRCA status with relatives (Hallowell et al. 2003). By becoming kin keepers and taking responsibility for the health of their families, these women often feel a sense of empowerment (Wilson and Etchegary 2010, 175). But with this new role comes the burden of deciding which relatives to tell, what specifically to disclose, and when the right time is to do it (Douglas, Hamilton, and Grubs 2009). Most women share the BRCA news with first-degree relatives, but telling extended relatives is often more difficult, especially when a woman is not particularly close to them—geographically or emotionally. It can strengthen bonds in families who will face cancer together, but sometimes causes unintended strife, so women are often selective about whom to share with (Claes et al. 2003).

Kim sent out letters to her family members to educate them about the BRCA mutation, share her positive result, and explain what generally follows the diagnosis.

> I have a science background . . . I'm used to having to explain all the science stuff, and medical stuff, to people in my family. So my, uh, my husband's side of the family has another inherited problem that I've had to explain to them, too. . . . When I sent them these letters, you know, I said, "Here are the current recommendations by the cancer society. It's get married, have your kids early, and then have the surgery done before the age of forty." And that's a lot to put on somebody.

Luckily, her family's reactions were generally positive. Kim says, "Cancer ran through our family like water through a sieve, so we were sort of glad to find out why." Sometimes BRCA information can actually be a relief to family members because it solves the mystery of their family's cancer history. Another woman said, "We were all relieved to know there was a reason behind it and that there were some things we could do proactively for it."

Some families react negatively to the messenger because they don't want to know their risk or to deal with genetic testing, cancer, and preventive surgeries. As Marla said about her own family: "I think they were maybe just in denial and didn't want anything to confirm that they might also be at risk . . . In fact, it's had a significant negative impact on the way I relate to my family, something I've struggled with since then." Many women feel they must do even more than simply tell their family members about their genetic risk—they must also influence them to act upon it through testing and preventive measures (Hallowell 1999). Such a proactive stance can fall flat if relatives aren't ready to think about health and mortality. Besides, the news of the BRCA mutation alone can cause psychological or emotional distress (Wilson and Etchegary 2010).

A BRCA-positive mutation diagnosis can take a toll on a woman even if she has a supportive family. She may feel guilty if the mutation is distributed unevenly among her relatives. Women negative for the BRCA mutation oftentimes feel survivor guilt for being lucky enough to escape the gene, and they struggle to watch loved ones who aren't so lucky (d'Agincourt-Canning 2006, 468). A similar guilt plagues some BRCA-positive women. Some women whose family members are diagnosed with cancer get tested and are able to prevent cancer for themselves. So while her relatives struggled with cancer, not knowing why and never having the change to prevent it, a BRCA-positive woman has the advantage of stopping cancer before it strikes. This advantage doesn't lessen the emotional trauma and struggles BRCA-positive women face, but many women feel guilty about these struggles that seem lesser than actually battling cancer. One woman described it in the following way.

> I feel a lot of guilt on a lot of different levels. Um, I have some guilt because right now I'm taking away so much from my family. Even though in the end I'm actually giving it back ten times over, you know? So I feel guilty as far as that. I feel guilty, you know, that my mom, you know, had cancer and all these other women have cancer, and I kind of got to cheat it, and I feel guilty, like survivor's guilt.

This sense of guilt can disempower women as they struggle to deal with their BRCA-positive status.

Let's not forget: men are part of the BRCA experience, too. But because breast cancer mostly affects women, it is more often women who educate their families about BRCA risk. They can also forget to tell their male relatives or lessen the importance of doing so. A BRCA club might form in BRCA-positive families, but men are often excluded, while women turn to each other for comfort and help making decisions. Men can struggle with BRCA as well, but gender can also keep men from seeking or accepting help. Women often pressure their brothers, nephews, uncles, or sons to get tested. Some men consider the risk of having a BRCA-positive mutation diagnosis to be just a woman's thing and dismiss it. As one woman described:

> There's certainly more of a stigma with women than men, but it's silly . . . I think it's more accepted that women have to find out their BRCA status because it seems as though it's more of a woman's problem than a man problem but it's really just as equally a man's problem. I think it's more of a social thing. I would think it's more of just the product of being a man . . . I don't think they think it's as big of a deal. They're not women, they don't have breasts, and they don't have ovaries, so why would this affect them?

Academics also focus on women's experiences and not men's. There is little scientific literature about men's decisions about BRCA testing (Hallowell et al. 2005). Even this book focuses specifically on women, although part of chapter 7 discusses men and the BRCA genetic testing experience. Although the BRCA mutation puts women at higher risk of cancer, it's important to acknowledge and look deeper at men's BRCA experiences as well. Men and women can rally together to fight their cancer risk.

Rallying the Family

Some women find strength and comfort in their families. They are empowered by following a path mapped out by their mother, aunts, or cousins who have already been diagnosed and made difficult decisions about prevention. Mothers can provide advice and support for daughters, and many women find unwavering strength in their partners. During hard times, this support is crucial for women to make confident and informed decisions.

For some women, a BRCA-positive mutation diagnosis is met with relief and strongly supportive family responses. There is an aha moment as relatives finally understand why such a strong history of cancer runs through the family. Knowing their status is knowledge that will rescue them from a fatal genetic destiny. One woman sharing her BRCA status can encourage information sharing within the entire family. A more detailed history of cancer develops and they realize how much can change thanks to genetic knowledge. They can even protect future generations from developing cancer.

A support network helps women as they handle the strain of BRCA on themselves and their families. Otherwise women would have to constantly defend their decisions and struggle with self-esteem (de Vries-Kragt 1998). Women with support from family members, friends, coworkers, and medical professionals are in a much better place psychologically to cope with a BRCA-positive mutation testing result. Many women, such as Emma, have incredible support systems in place.

Emma is a married woman in her early forties. She comes from a long line of women who have had breast cancer, a family history she calls "abysmal." Her grandmother died from it, her mother and twin sister are breast cancer survivors, and, like Emma, the latter are both BRCA positive. Perhaps because of this history and its emotional toll, Emma has had support from everyone in her life: her husband, her three children, her mother and twin sister, her church, even her entire neighborhood.

> My daughters, my husband, and son and I and all of us have always talked about the risk, you know. Um, we all felt like it was, it was what we should do, what I should do. And yeah, I had the support of everyone that they would do what they could to help and all that. . . . Every single person I've talked to in my family, friends, church, everywhere has said, "You have a great chance." . . . [My husband] said, obviously whatever we need to do to protect your life. And that's what everybody said, too. Complete, complete support . . . It's been a really good support, too, because all of the people that I know in this neighborhood, which, I mean there are 200 people . . . have said, "You're doing the right thing." You know, and, "We'll support you."

Emma has stayed positive and happy with no regrets about her BRCA-related decisions.

The BRCA experience often brings family closer together in the struggle against cancer. Cynthia is a forty-five-year-old Ashkenazi Jewish woman whose mother, daughter, and sister all have the BRCA mutation. When she tested positive as well, Cynthia immediately had her ovaries removed because she was afraid she, too, would develop cancer. Even while recovering from this preventive surgery, Cynthia cared for another sister who was in the last stages of her breast cancer.

Despite the devastating loss of her sister, Cynthia has remained positive throughout her own experience. One reason is the strong emotional support she receives from her husband of thirty years. As she tells it, prior to her BRCA diagnosis they had a supportive and loving relationship. They are both psychologists and in the field of marital counseling, so they are well aware that poor communication can destroy a marriage. She and her husband approach her BRCA experience with a sense of camaraderie and humor.

> I'm very blessed. I have a very, um, open, loving, accepting relationship with my spouse . . . I feel like through this whole process my relationship with my husband has gotten, um, even more—we've gotten, um, the intimacy has gotten even stronger. . . . We didn't wait very long at all [to have sex after I removed my breasts]. When I came home from the hospital, I had surgical drains and stuff, but he still wanted to make love. And it was really good that we did, because it was such a life-affirming, and it was like getting back in the saddle and realizing, yeah, you know, I'm still the same, and we're still the same. And even with all these tubes attached to me, it's still great. And that was great.

The couple realized early on the need to create a new normal in their post–BRCA and post–surgical life (this idea of a new normal is the topic of chapter 7). Because her husband has to deal with some difficult health issues himself, he is particularly empathic about her illness. Seeing her sister die made it clear to Cynthia, her husband, and their family that staying alive is the number one priority. So sharing her BRCA results was not a problem for Cynthia, who sees the news as important to all family members. It's something to be discussed and addressed. She didn't try to hide it from anyone, and she feels comfortable in her BRCA status and about her later surgical decisions.

When Cynthia was tested for the BRCA mutation, her daughter Isabelle was in her teens. Part of her upbeat attitude then, she notes, was her desire to be a positive role model for her daughter, who had not yet been tested. Isabelle has since tested positive, but Cynthia tries to stay upbeat to create a sense of normalcy for her daughter. She is trying to shield her child from the difficult decisions ahead.

Isabelle herself says that being tested at such a young age changed her life and her family. When she first learned about her risk of being a BRCA carrier, she put the issue on the back burner. She was more worried about her mother's preventive surgeries and her aunt's condition than about herself. Isabelle eventually did get tested. She remembers learning the news as a "very detached moment." It took her many months to process. Instead, she focused on moving to a new state and seeking employment. She notes:

> I wasn't consciously like, "Okay, what am I going to do? What does this mean? What's my future?" I just wanted to kind of put it aside in my mind, so I could get ready to move and . . . start my new job. I'd just finished grad school, figured out, you know, what I was going to do with my career, find a boyfriend, um, you know, make friends, girl-friends, and figure out the city. There was so much other stuff that was going through my mind that I really wasn't putting it in the forefront.

When Isabelle started dating post-testing, she struggled with sharing her BRCA status. It was easy to disclose if she didn't think she had a future with them. There was nothing to lose. But it was harder when she started to date her future husband. She waited four months, waiting until things became "more serious." She was nervous but sure about telling him.

> I was confident enough that the person I would pick would be accepting of it and would love me for who I am. . . . There was a little part of me that was worried, like, maybe it is too much or maybe even though he's an accepting person maybe he's not mature enough to handle it. . . . But he was able to handle it.

Sharing her BRCA status can be challenging but ultimately it can bring people closer together.

Like many young BRCA-positive mutation carriers, Isabelle felt pressured to have children, although she took her time to find the right husband, a topic that is covered more fully in chapters 4 and 5. Isabelle's doctors encouraged her to have children before age thirty-six. She was trying to become pregnant at the time of our interview, and hoped to have at least two children before she "needed" to have preventive surgery. Isabelle and Cynthia's stories paint a positive picture of the ways family members can work together to address familial cancer risk. But all women's stories are not as happy.

Disrupting Family Dynamics

Every woman's relationships or perspective on family changed in some way once they shared their BRCA-positive status. For better or for worse, a BRCA-positive mutation diagnosis changes families. And family members don't always support one another when someone shares the BRCA news. One of the most challenging situations for a family is when more than one family member gets tested but they have different results. When Tara and her sisters were tested for BRCA, only her results came back positive. Combined with disagreement about Tara's preventive decisions, BRCA has strained her relationships with her sisters. They "totally" withdrew from her after learning she was positive. She is frustrated that they don't support her surgical decision. Because her mother is also BRCA positive and has supported Tara, they have forged a special bond that further alienates her sisters.

> My sisters and people around didn't understand [my mother's decision to get a mastectomy]. But I was proud of her because it was taking her—her life into her own hands instead of just waiting for something to happen to her. . . . Not that they're jealous, but maybe a jealousy that my mom have that in common to share, because you know, just with sisters there's always a rivalry and always competing for the parents' attention.

It's hard to understand the BRCA testing and positive mutation diagnosis experience unless you've lived it. Tara wants to tell BRCA-negative people, "Don't tell me what I'm doing is wrong because it's my body and it's my decision."

Some families clash when different generations hold different values about getting tested. Individuals and cultures might not value genetic knowledge at all. June, who was mentioned earlier, is of Chinese descent and is at odds with her family. She has found that cultural barriers to genetic testing and disclosure run deep in her traditional family. Her parents, both born in China and now living in the United States, don't agree with the American preventive medical model. "It's like [my parents] don't believe in finding out," June explains. "So they just believe in fate, you know? . . . [In]

China they don't have that kind of testing. They don't believe in that. Not like here in the U.S., you know?" June has had no success in reaching out to her family about getting tested: "When I told my parents that I was positive, I kind of wanted to see if my sister was interested in finding out, or if my mom was interested," but they "didn't do anything." She attributes this disinterest partially to traditional Chinese culture.

> I would say they like to let nature take its course. . . . Like, if it's going to happen, it's gonna happen. You don't do anything to prevent it. They just don't want to deal with it until it happens. . . . Knowing the information is good to them. But they think that after knowing that information, I could utilize that information and take care of myself in terms of my daily lifestyle [and not by getting preventive surgery].

When she told her parents she was positive, they "just hushed it away." June is struggling without their support to get preventive surgery. Family support is crucial to making these medical decisions. "I think it would help me a lot if I had family support, that they'd agree with my decision," she says. "I think that's very traditional in [a] Chinese family, [but] if you can't get everybody to agree with you, it's kinda hard, you know?" As you learn in chapter 4, June's and her parents' relationship remains strained.

Women's relationships with their husbands or significant others can also become strained. In the worst cases, BRCA can end a relationship altogether. Andrea calls her BRCA diagnosis "a wake up" to the reality of her poor relationship with her husband. His inability to be there for her made her realize she "didn't have time to waste" on him. She asked for a divorce after twenty-three years of marriage. Andrea explains, "Your perspective just so changes, you know? I mean, what if I was going to die in five years? This is not . . . I'm not gonna waste five years more." Andrea's diagnosis was "a gift" and not a worst-case scenario at all.

The same is not true for Erica and her husband. Their relationship changed but it hasn't ended after she learned the news and got preventive surgery.

> The relationship changed significantly, to be honest. For me, the inability to really talk about what was going on at a deep level kind of disconnected me from him emotionally. . . . We still live in the same house, and we're with the kids and we have fun together, but for me, um, I wouldn't still be married if I didn't have two young kids, to be bluntly

honest . . . I needed the emotional support. I needed the mutual interest in learning about the condition. And I needed more conversation
about the future.

Erica feels unsupported by her husband. He can't "just sit down and talk
about the fears involved with finding out" and he refuses to address real-
istically their inability to pay their increasing medical bills. Because of this
experience, her marriage will never be the same.

Erica also feels a new distance from her parents and extended family.
When she explained her BRCA-positive status to them, what she remembers
most is silence: "I talked to my sister a little bit, and then no one in the family talked to me for about two months. . . . It was like they were afraid and
they didn't want to hear the word 'cancer' and they didn't want to know that
it was hereditary." Her parents' fear of cancer is so strong that, at the time of
the interview, they had not spoken to her in two months. Erica comments,
"What's interesting is that two weeks after my mastectomy, when my parents
were here, they left. . . . That was the end of October, [and] my parents have
not called me since." Some families succumb to shock and fear for their own
well-being. It can prevent them from supporting those who have already
tested positive. Families can fall apart.

"I think they're afraid of losing me, [but] in an odd way they've lost me."

Learning the News Early On: Young BRCA-Positive Women

A woman's age—and her place along life's journey—has a signficant impact
on how she reacts to learning the news. Women are being tested at younger
and younger ages because both the information about and the availability
of genetic testing have increased. As we saw in Isabelle's story earlier, young
women with the BRCA mutation who are just starting out their lives may
feel pressured to change their life plans for children or marriage to address
their cancer risk. These young women have to figure out a timeline for their
futures so that BRCA doesn't overshadow their other life goals.

One of the primary concerns for a young, unmarried woman with a
BRCA-positive mutation result is its effect on her ability to have a family. Especially with preventive surgery as an option, many women are torn
between removing their breasts or ovaries to prevent cancer and delaying
preventive surgery in order to have children. One woman described it:

I wanted to get pregnant, and I wanted to breast-feed. My doctor told me that it's actually better after you've had a full-term pregnancy, um, because there's more tissues down there. So, you kind of, interestingly, getting, finding these test results is what lit a fire under my butt to have a family . . . I thought, "Well if I'm going to get rid of my female organs, I want to use them first." And so, I got pregnant and I had a baby.

Many women try to beat the cancer clock. Some are pressured to get pregnant before their preventive surgeries but prioritize their health. Another woman was happy to get tested after deciding not to have children. She explains, "I'm like, wow, that's great, I didn't pass my genetics on to somebody. Let's stop here."

Young women also worry how this diagnosis will affect them in the dating world. Hereditary genetic mutations and high cancer risk are not easy topics to bring up, even with loved ones of many years. It's difficult to decide the right time and way to share their BRCA status and to be prepared for the possibility of rejection. Many women become resolved to find a life partner who could potentially support them through preventive surgeries and decision making (Werner-Lin 2008). But they also consider how surgery will affect their attractiveness, whether a partner can handle the fear of cancer, and the potential medical bills. A partner's reaction to the BRCA news can be a test of the relationship itself; if it was meant to last, then it will (Klitzman and Sweeney 2011). Women want to communicate the seriousness of BRCA while downplaying it at the same time so they don't frighten a partner (Hoskins et al. 2008).

Even in a serious relationship, disclosing her positive status can be difficult. After all, this puts a lot of pressure on her partner, too. All sorts of questions will leap to mind. How can I support her? Will we be able to have children together? Do we have to start planning our family right away? What will I do if we fall out of love just as she gets sick? Carrie wonders how BRCA affects her relationships with her boyfriend.

He was very supportive of me going to get screening. For years, he always wanted me to get tested. But, in a way, I was always hesitant because it scared me to, like, find out the results and how it would almost impact us, you know, and the pressure it would put on us. . . . We're in a conflicted part, because he gets it, and he wants to be there for me, but, at the same time, I don't necessarily expect him to change, like, his life and what he's ready for just because of this news.

Changing two people's life plans and goals is a challenge for young couples that receive the BRCA-positive mutation diagnosis news. One partner's health status can create tension in the relationship. Carrie continues:

I plan on having the surgery sometime in the very near future. And he's very supportive, and he wants me to have it. You know, the thought of me not having it really upsets him, you know. . . . Like, I'm confident 100% that, if I have the surgery, he'll be here with me when I need him to be there. But whether he's with me for the long run is a whole other story.

Carrie has the doubts of any normal relationship but with the additional pressure of BRCA and the threat of cancer. Despite the challenges, she thinks that surgery could strengthen her connection with her boyfriend: "With him I would obviously hope it would bring us closer, you know, because it would be much more of an emotional connection. . . . We are beyond the physical, I think, to some degree." In the meantime, she continues to try to maintain a sense of normalcy.

Getting tested for the BRCA mutation is only a step to further decisions: who to tell of their positive status, who to depend on for support, how to assess their cancer risk, and what all this means for their decisions about cancer prevention. Surgical decisions are based on how women assess their risk of getting cancer, which I discuss further in chapter 4. With a positive BRCA result comes at least one inevitable choice: surgery or surveillance? What options are available to these women, and how viable are hey for women at different points in their lives? Will their families support these decisions? For young women, what does a positive test result mean for future family planning and relationships? And for older women, what are the risks associated with preventive surgery or with increased surveillance? We continue to follow the journey of BRCA-positive women and see how they answer these questions.

FOUR

Waiting and Watching

I came to be tested because my mother actually was diagnosed with breast cancer about four years ago, and she was only forty-five, and so they were kind of already a little bit concerned. And then it came out that two of her aunts and two of her cousins, all on the same side of the family, all had breast cancer at a fairly young age, so they tested her. She was positive for, um, BRCA2. And so then, you know, it was kind of agreed that I would test when I was closer to being twenty-five because they, apparently they don't start additional surveillance until you're at least twenty-five. . . . So they were kind of like, "If you don't want to test yet, there's no real need to." They wouldn't do anything differently either way.

I'd been planning on this for almost four years. . . . In all honesty, I had kind of always assumed it would be positive for some reason, so I just figured, it's probably better to get tested and then I can start with the surveillance, and, you know, make sure I can prevent cancer. And I don't know if that—I don't know if there was necessarily a reason for it, I always just assumed that would be the case. And I don't know if that was just me kind of having a doomsday scenario, or if it was partially just because I had heard so much about it. Because my mom had gone through the whole thing, I watched my mom go through all the surgeries and all of the, you know, everything related to her cancer.

[Some people's] mentality is just: "I'm going to do everything I can right now to avoid getting cancer because I want, you know, to beat it before it even can—before I even have it." And I do absolutely agree with that, I just don't personally feel that [surgery is] something I need to do right this minute. You know, when I'm talking to doctors and they're telling me that, you know, the likelihood of me getting cancer right now is very, very low, even though I do have this gene mutation, I don't feel that I need to, you know, instantly uproot my entire life, spend all this time in the hospital having surgery, recovering from surgery, when it's probably okay if I wait a few years and do it then.

Holly is young and dealing with her BRCA-positive mutation status, facing the emotional highs and lows, making the difficult decisions about surveillance and surgery. She has always assumed she'll be diagnosed with cancer. She's done a lot of research and one day she may get a mastectomy and oophorectomy, but for now she is content with regular surveillance.

Erin's experience was a bit different. She recalls returning to the genetic clinic to get her results. At first, she thought all would be well. After all, her counselor greeted her warmly, with a big smile. Then she heard the words that would change her life forever: "We've got your results, and you tested positive for BRCA1 mutation." For the first few weeks after that, she was fine. In fact, she only remembered what had been discussed in her counseling session because of the handout she was given. But questions about her future came crashing down on her when her family doctor, in a follow-up appointment, said, "Let's talk about when you would like your ovaries removed." She was just thirty-four, unmarried, and not in a steady relationship. What to do?

The next two chapters explore this question. Like deciding whether to be tested or to disclose your results, deciding what steps to take after receiving a positive result is a process—one that is highly complex and often revisited. A woman will think and think again about a host of possibilities as she assesses her cancer risk and reaches out to others—family and friends, doctors and other experts—through her social, medical, and online networks. She will also investigate her family's cancer history in order to estimate her actual risk, and she will use this knowledge to weigh treatment options.

After receiving a BRCA-positive mutation result, a woman can choose from many paths. Some women have decided what course to take even before they get the test; others are suddenly motivated by their results to take action. Overall, though, the choice seems to be between two general directions: surgery or surveillance? Some women make this choice immediately after getting their results, while others weigh their options. Still more women will go in one direction initially and change course to adapt to changing circumstances. A woman might, for example, choose surveillance until she has a child—and then decide to have her ovaries removed.

No matter what general path she takes, however, she can be empowered or disempowered by her experience. And the next two chapters investigate why. They also consider how a woman decides between surveillance, surgery, or some combination of the two and who and what affect her decisions.

But first, we need to understand how BRCA-positive mutation women assess their risk for cancer. We see that family, family medical history, and medical statistics all influence a woman's determination of her risk. The rest of this chapter focuses specifically on women who choose the surveillance option, while the next discusses women who choose preventative surgery. When women who have a high risk of breast and ovarian cancer opt for surveillance, they monitor the health of their breasts and ovaries and make regular medical appointments in order to screen for cancer. The idea is to detect the disease as early as possible. Screening methods for breast cancer are mammograms and physical breast exams, either done by a woman herself or by her health-care provider. Any irregularities in a mammogram can be followed up through magnetic resonance imaging (MRI) or biopsy. Surveillance for ovarian cancer tends to be more challenging, involving transvaginal ultrasounds or blood tests. So whether a woman is at high risk for ovarian cancer (because she is BRCA1 rather than BRCA2 positive) can affect dramatically whether she opts for surveillance or surgery. In any event, assessing cancer risk is crucial.

Calculating the Odds

What exactly does a BRCA-positive mutation result mean? When a woman learns she is BRCA positive, and sometimes long before then, she must determine her risk for cancer. And it's rarely as simple as listening to the numbers her doctor says.

Beyond sharing the information with her family, one of the most important processes women go through after getting a positive BRCA result is to assess their risk of getting breast or ovarian cancer. Doctors, nurses, and genetics counselors are the first, usually, to begin explaining what a woman's BRCA test results mean in terms of her risk for getting cancer. To communicate, they use the statistical language of cancer-risk models based on large population samples. But the medical risk is the same for all women who test positive: each has a lifetime risk (based on a life expectancy of eighty-five years) of developing breast cancer that ranges from 60 to 90 percent for BRCA1 and 30 to 85 percent for BRCA2 (National Cancer Institute 2009).

Often, women who are BRCA positive recall encountering an unstated assumption amongst those who counsel them about risk—that all women will interpret these numbers in accordance with current medical opinion and take expert advice about what treatment they should undergo because of their high-risk cancer status. But the women in my study interpret this news in many different ways. They have individual responses to the information, and unique answers to the main questions arising from that information: What does it means to be "at high risk" for cancer? How should I think about this? What actions, if any, should I take as preventative measures against cancer?

Medical providers and genetics counselors are often the first people who help a woman interpret her results. They're there to deliver the news and help explain what a positive result means. Providers tend to use statistical language based on medical models that result from studying large populations. Because these numbers are based on large populations and not an individual's unique circumstances, the statistical medical risk is the same for all women who test positive. Women in the general population have a 12 percent risk of developing breast cancer and 1.2 percent risk of ovarian cancer in their lifetime (based on a life expectancy of eighty-five years). Being diagnosed with the BRCA1 or BRCA2 gene mutations raise their breast cancer risk to 60 percent and ovarian cancer risk to 15–40 percent (National Cancer Institute 2009). But even these statistics can waver, depending on the source, as BRACAnalysis®'s commercial website claims that a BRCA-positive woman's risk of breast cancer by age seventy is 56–87 percent, and of ovarian cancer is 15–44 percent (National Cancer Institute, 2012).

The most important thing to understand, however, is that each woman filters the meaning of being BRCA-positive mutation diagnosis through the lens of her own lived experiences. She considers her family relationships, as well as her connections to those outside her family network. For example, did she grow up in family where there was a strong history of cancer? Did she lose a loved one to breast or ovarian cancer—a mother, an aunt, or a cousin? If there was no history of any cancer in her family while she was growing up, did *she* have a cancer scare? Was she diagnosed with cancer before she got tested? If so, she will interpret the meaning of a positive diagnosis through the lens of her own experience with cancer. Because women construct their own risk assessment through these lived experiences, they almost always perceive their risk to be significantly higher than it actually is. And a woman's perception of her risk rather than her actual risk is more important in determining what she decides to do next (Tambor, Rimer, and

Strigo 1997; Zikmund-Fisher, Fagerlin, and Ubel 2010). Why? Our perceptions are rooted in our emotions, in our memories of and reactions to events. And strong emotional experiences trump statistical information any day, which my study demonstrated.

The point in her life at which a woman learns the news also influences her risk assessment: Is she just starting off her life as a young single woman? Is she married or in a significant relationship? Is she contented in that relationship? Is she divorced or widowed? Does she have children? Does she want more children? These life circumstances help make up a rich and diverse relational context, one unique to each woman. And each interprets her positive BRCA, mutation result within that context.

To assess their risk of cancer, the women I interviewed do not necessarily rely on the statistical models provided by medical professionals. Rather, they base their assessments from the hot spots in the cancer histories of their own families. Was an aunt diagnosed with breast cancer at age forty? Did an older sister die from ovarian cancer at fifty-nine? Sometimes, these age markers become like magical numbers that a woman imposes on her own life cycle. By looking at the multigenerational stories of her extended family, a BRCA-positive woman can use her family's cancer clock as a strong guide to assess her own odds of developing cancer—and to calibrate how much time she has before she must do something. Family narratives simultaneously provide a sense of guidance through the process of addressing BRCA and a connection to a woman's family (Werner-Lin and Gardner 2009).

Natalie is twenty-eight years old and single. She tested positive for the BRCA mutation six months prior to our interview. She based her decisions about prevention upon her mother's experiences. Her mother was first diagnosed with breast cancer at thirty-one. So, as Natalie explains, she is "planning to do the prophylactic mastectomy, um, certainly before I'm thirty." Originally, she was tested only because her mother was diagnosed with cancer for a second time. Because of her close relationship with her mother, Natalie finds comfort in using her mother's experience as a guide to help her fight cancer successfully. Especially because she "doesn't really know her family history" of cancer, her mother's lived experiences are crucial to her current decisions.

Christina (we met her in chapter 3) saw the challenge she faced in determining what her risk really was. And it was the numbers that pushed her over the edge to choose surgery. She said, "What really convinced me [to get surgery] is the 40–85 percent statistic. And when a doctor tells you something like that, you aren't thinking, 'Oh, maybe my risk is 40 percent.' No.

Like [laughing], your risk is 85 percent. Some of the doctors told me, you know, with my family history, it's 90 percent." When one medical technician said she thought prophylactic surgery was extreme, Christina responded, "Did you not hear me when I said 90 percent chance of cancer?" Clearly, Christina leaned toward the higher estimate when it came to her own risk.

Medical professionals usually assume women will go by the statistical risk they provide. They expect a woman to interpret these numbers as her actual risk and act according to her doctor's suggested treatment protocol. But when you listen to a woman's story, it's easy to see that their doctor's recommendations are only a part of determining their own risk. Once they consider a wide range of personal factors, a woman may think that her risk is as high as 100 percent. And her decisions about preventive care can stray even further from a doctor's recommendations. This is especially true because some doctors will advocate for prophylactic surgery while others would almost never recommend it, especially for a younger woman. The medical community itself isn't even consistent in its recommendations to women. It is impossible to predict what a woman will say is her own risk for cancer, but most women's stories follow a similar pattern.

A woman interprets her BRCA-positive mutation results and cancer risk based on her own lived experiences. She especially considers her family's history. Did she grow up in family where there was a strong history of cancer? Has she lost loved ones to breast or ovarian cancer—her mother, aunt, or cousin? Was she diagnosed with cancer herself? A woman who doesn't learn she is BRCA positive until after a cancer diagnosis may have an even greater sense of her risk of recurrence. These kinds of personal and family experiences will usually heighten a woman's fear of cancer and raise her perceived risk above what her doctors tell her. My follow-up small on-line survey of the sixty-four women I interviewed said that after getting their positive results, they felt their risk of getting cancer on average was 82.3 percent. And how a woman feels is more important than statistical risk to her decisions about prevention (Tambor, Rimer, and Strigo 1997; Zikmund-Fisher, Fagerlin, and Ubel 2010).

A woman's risk takes on relative weight depending on where she is on her life's path. Is she a young unmarried woman? Is she married or in a committed relationship? Does she have children? The answers to these question can make addressing her risk for cancer more or less important and may make her interpret her risk are higher or lower. These many factors create a rich context in which a woman creates her own meaning of her BRCA-positive mutation result.

Christina is like many women who base their risk on the course of cancer in their family members' lives. Christina always assumed her diagnosis would come at the same age as her mother's. She said, "I figured the thirties were when it was going to strike me, you know, it seemed like it was going down a decade every generation, so that really helped make my decision to do it as soon as I did." These ages at which a woman's family was diagnosed with cancer become magical numbers in predicting her own future. Multiple cases of cancer in a family can allow women to even better—in their opinion—predict when cancer will come. Looking at the history of cancer and BRCA-positive mutation results throughout the generations tells them how much time they have before they must do something. A woman's family narrative also gives her guidance and often a support system when addressing their BRCA-positive mutation status (Werner-Lin and Gardner 2009).

Another woman, Kelsey, also made decisions about prevention by looking at her mother's experiences. Her mother was first diagnosed with breast cancer at thirty-one, so Kelsey explains she is "planning to do the prophylactic mastectomy, um, certainly before I'm thirty." Originally, she was only tested because her mother was diagnosed with cancer for a second time. Because of her close relationship with her mother, Kelsey finds comfort in using her mother's experience as a guide in order to successfully fight against cancer. Especially because she "doesn't really know her family history" of cancer, her mother's lived experiences are especially crucial to her current decision making.

> My mom's cancer was, even though I don't remember and my brother was really young, it's always been a really big part of our lives. . . . My mom's history doesn't give me a whole lot of information as far as decision-making with all of this . . . I don't want to get cancer. Like that's the bottom line. Um, so I'm planning to do the prophylactic mastectomy, certainly before I'm thirty. But possibly even earlier than that. I want to be around, and I don't want to get cancer.

Placing Bets on Waiting

Her risk of cancer is just one of many things a woman considers when deciding what steps to take after getting her BRCA-positive mutation result. Just like the difficult decision about even getting tested, a woman's decision about prevention is influenced by many factors related to her life stage and the people in her life. Research on medical decision making often assumes that BRCA-positive mutation women follow a specific protocol that relies on health-care providers' expert knowledge in order to decide on a plan of action (Forde 1998; Glanz, Rimer, and Lewis 2002; Rodney et al. 2004). Much of the research assumes that when women learn their risk, they should go with the recommendations of medical providers and authorities (Pilarski 2009). As I mentioned earlier in this chapter, women generally choose between surveillance and surgery to prevent cancer, but women's decisions are not so straightforward (Hopwood et al. 2000; Lerman et al. 2000; Metcalfe and Narod 2002). So what makes a woman decide on surveillance?

For most, surveillance is actually a given. Based on my follow up online survey of the sixty-four BRCA-positive mutation women I interviewed, most women who carry the BRCA mutation gene (78.6 percent) will elect surveillance at some point in their lives, whether before or after the test, and including women who later go on to get prophylactic surgery. Women often have an idea of their cancer risk without the BRCA test and will get regular cancer screenings throughout their life. Even after finding out they're BRCA-positive mutation carriers, many women feel that preventive surgery—especially a mastectomy, more so than an oophorectomy—is too drastic. For at least some part of their lives, a woman is willing to wait for cancer to come while choosing surveillance methods that will catch it early. At the same time, research shows that 65 percent of BRCA-positive women think it's the best way to reduce the risk and worry of breast cancer (Litton et al. 2009). So because women see surveillance as not wholly effective, it's not usually a lifelong course that BRCA-positive mutation women take in order to combat their risk of cancer. Most women who start with surveillance eventually get prophylactic surgery as well, which I discuss in chapter 5.

Health-care providers certainly play an important role in women's decisions to have surveillance. Many women will elect to have an oophorectomy if their family is complete, but will continue monitoring their breasts for cancer. There are many reasons to put off a mastectomy: avoiding a painful, lengthy, and unnecessary surgery and recovery; financial costs; wanting natural breasts; wanting to breastfeed. One woman was torn but followed this path for various reasons, including her painful childhood memories of her mother's mastectomy. She was also calmed by her doctor's support for surveillance.

When I go into see my, um, breast doctor, you know, I guess about every other time, I say, "Are you sure we don't need to have my breasts removed?" And he keeps reassuring me, "I am telling you, everything we are doing, if you get cancer, we will catch it so early, SO early, you are not going to have to—you are not going to die—you are not going to have to be worried about this. It's going to be so early."

For good or bad, doctors can encourage a woman to continue surveillance, even when she has doubts as to whether it is the best decision for her.

Most women who choose surveillance tend to share one important thing in common: no one close to them has died of cancer. Not a single woman in my study who opted for surveillance had any close family member die of cancer. Something about the experience of watching a loved one die of cancer seems to push women to have prophylactic surgery to avoid that experience themselves. Research shows that the main reason women choose preventive surgery is to take aggressive action against the cancer that killed a family member (Hamilton et al. 2009). Women who have not lost a loved one to cancer do not feel that same need to eradicate the fear of cancer entirely. They don't see themselves with as high a risk and more often choose surveillance. Later in this chapter we hear Olivia's story. She shows us the importance of family history in this decision—that is, a woman with little to no family history is more likely to not choose preventive surgery. We also hear June's story and see how her family actively pushed her away from surveillance, even against her own wishes.

Women who choose surveillance are also younger, unmarried, and child-less. Understandable, when prophylactic surgery can pose so many challenges: prevent breastfeeding or childbearing, launch a woman into early menopause, and more. The women I spoke with who had chosen surveillance at the time we spoke were, on average, thirty-five years old (vs. age thirty-nine of all women). Half were unmarried (vs. 28.6 percent of women who chose preventive surgery) and most didn't have children at the time (only 35.7 percent had at least one child, compared to 57.1 percent of women who elected preventive surgery). Research has also found that younger women are more likely to commit to regular mammograms (Isaacs et al. 2002; De Leeuw, van Vliet, and Ausems 2008). These younger women feel they have more time and freedom to plan for the future before cancer might develop. In chapter 5, I go into more detail about these and other reasons that women delay preventive surgery.

Olivia and June's stories give us some insight into how women can feel empowered—or not—by their surveillance decision. When a woman chooses surveillance as a proactive treatment option, she generally feels empowered. She has made her peace with her BRCA-positive status. Women sometimes take on a type of fatalistic attitude that they accept as part of who they are. As one woman noted, "We are a fix it up culture and sometimes, we can't fix things. . . . If cancer comes, it comes." But this isn't the case for everyone. Some women seem to choose surveillance by default because they lack support from family and friends for choosing surgery. They might just not have the support or resources to make an informed decision. It's not even that easy to say whether a woman's decision is empowering or not.

Empowerment is "a process of change" that allows women to feel they can "shape their own lives" (Narayan 2005, 72, 4). In this book, I describe surveillance as empowering for women if they're content with their decision and receive the support they need, whether simply in themselves or from family and friends. Women often say that knowledge is power when it comes to the BRCA testing and positive mutation diagnosis experience. As one woman described:

> Knowledge is power. It sucks, but then you realize you're in control. You can be in as much control as you can be. And that's not to say that everyone should go get a prophylactic mastectomy. For me that was the right decision. But women can go get more preventative screenings. A lot of times, people are sitting ducks. And I understand, to go get tested is a very big thing, but it's just how you view it. I entered it kind of naively and I came out a lot more knowledgeable

So having the time and ability to seek out information about her options is also empowering. Most women will do a lot of their own research online. They might even reach out to more than one provider to get different opinions. The amount of information available can be overwhelming, and finding credible sources of information can be frustrating, but the process allows women to make more informed decisions (Babb et al. 2002). The search for this information is for many women an empowering act in itself because it allows them to have a hand in their own destiny.

Being empowered often comes down to the simple feeling of being in control. A woman is empowered when she knows that the decision is hers and that she is doing the best she can to face her risk of cancer. Women undergoing surveillance often consider preventive surgery as an option for the future, but for now they have time to pursue other life choices like marriage and children before changing their decision. Studies have shown that women have a better sense of their quality of life, and feel more empowered, when they feel they are more involved in their making their own decisions after the BRCA test (Andersen et al. 2009).

Yet a woman can be disempowered in choosing surveillance if it's not the choice she really wants to make. Later in this chapter, we hear June's story and see how some women are conflicted about a surgical decision that feels right but violates their family's values and wishes. If a woman's family is unsupportive, then having alternative networks of social support, including friends and contacts online, is vital to making empowered decisions. Some women simply live in denial of their BRCA-positive status. They go with surveillance and push their fear to the back of their minds, assuming it doesn't have to be dealt with, at least not yet.

In the next two sections, Olivia and June tell their stories and their lived experiences with surveillance. Their decisions follow completely different paths when it comes to surveillance. Olivia is very empowered, and June is very unhappy. Let's hear why.

Olivia's Story: Placing Bets on Watching

I think that I hadn't really wrapped my mind around [the test]. It is sort of something that I did. I think that's what makes it unusual for me, because I haven't had somebody close to me have breast cancer and kinda had to think about this all through my life. So, um, I was surprised that, um, how badly I felt. I just felt like it would be something that happens, it would probably be negative, it's a fifty-fifty chance. For some reason I didn't think that I would have it. Even though I know probabilities well. I think I've been significantly down. More down this month.

Olivia is a white, single woman in her thirties. She doesn't feel like the test was really her decision, or at least not something she fully thought through. Perhaps this is because she doesn't have much of a family history of cancer—only her grandfather is a breast cancer survivor. Both her grandfather and her father were tested for the BRCA1 and BRCA2 gene mutations before her, and both tested positive.

When Olivia first learned about the test, she waited about a year as she finished her Ph.D program, but was tested before taking on the time commitment of a position at a prestigious university. At the time we spoke, Olivia had found out she was BRCA-positive mutation carrier, just one month prior. Before getting the test, Olivia didn't fully consider her options for prevention. She had no set plan in mind in the case that she tested positive. So when she received the surprisingly results, she felt "significantly down" and as she learned more and more about what it means to be a BRCA-positive mutation carrier, she felt even worse.

Olivia never even considered prophylactic surgery until her genetic counselor brought it up. She learned from the counselor that 50 percent of BRCA-positive women elect prophylactic mastectomy and even more remove their ovaries after age forty. Olivia reflected on this but easily decided not to have preventive surgery.

> At first I was very unsure. I shouldn't say at first, because this is still very early. But I'm fairly confident now that, um, I'm not going to have, um, definitely not the prophylactic. I shouldn't say definitely not, but not the prophylactic double mastectomy. It's just not, um, it's just not my approach, I think, to life I guess, I don't know. It just doesn't seem like something I could . . . I know people feel it's empowering. To me it doesn't feel empowering to . . . take such a drastic measure. I feel it's kind of fearful, and unnatural . . . I'm not sure about removing my ovaries. I think that I have a decade before I decide that, and I think that even that I'm very apprehensive about.

Olivia is dedicated to better surveillance, but undecided about getting mammograms because of the radiation. Instead, she has opted for MRIs, which she now qualifies for under her health insurance because of her positive BRCA result.

Olivia feels time is still on her side and surveillance means she doesn't have to worry about cancer. She also attributes her surveillance decision to the fact that she has not seen somebody close to her die of cancer.

> I think the fact that I haven't seen somebody die close to me of cancer might be affecting my decision. But I read the stories online, um, of women who are making these decisions. And, um, in a lot of cases, if you've seen your mother die of cancer, I think you're just willing to— it's closer to home. Or just even suffering of cancer. Anything. You might want to be more aggressive in preventing that outcome. Um, but even though I know that, I still can't. I know that there's no reason to think that I'm at any less risk than they are. I feel it's very difficult to justify, even with an 85 percent probability.

Because no one in her family has died of cancer, and her grandfather's experience seemed so mild, her decision "not to do anything" is easier to make.

As I noted earlier, family history of cancer is vital to women's decision making about surveillance and surgery. The stories that Olivia has read online about women who choose surgery make her think that women who have seen their mothers die of cancer might be more willing to have preventive surgery because cancer is "closer to home."

From the stories she has read, Olivia thinks that women who choose surgeries while young are "actively deciding not just to wait to get cancer, but to avoid it, to prevent it." But Olivia looks at her BRCA-positive mutation status from a different viewpoint.

> I feel like embracing what's going to happen, accepting risks, and not altering my body so dramatically is another way to be empowered . . . I think it's very brave to go through the surgery, and I don't think I'm fearful of surgery. I really don't think that that's the reason . . . I think the largest part is [that] I don't feel that I would want to take such drastic measures to sort of alter my health path when I'm healthy now. I think that we do a lot of things in our lives that change our risk of life and death. And I think that, um, I'm just accepting that this is my body and this is, I'm going to be healthy, behave healthfully, and not do anything active to shorten my life. But I'm not going to, at the same time, because of this potential, um, for me to get cancer or in forty years, also drastically alter my body.

She accepts some additional risk in choosing surveillance, knowing "potentially how I'm going to die." But surveillance is a reasonable choice to make in the face of that risk, and she sees no point in "drastically" altering her body with preventive surgery.

Olivia gets much strength in choosing surveillance from the support of her family and friends who have helped her make this decision. In particular, her mother pointed out to Olivia that preventive surgery didn't fit her usual mode of addressing problems; that she isn't the kind of person who would "remove body parts" in order to simply fix the problem and try to make it go away. Olivia appreciated her mother's support as well as her boyfriend's. He was especially helpful with doing research and opening her eyes to the wider context—like we discussed in chapter 1—in which women make decisions about surgery.

Doing research on her own made the decision all the more empowering. Olivia was able to see the choices of surveillance and surgery from a broader perspective. She realized there were forces bigger than her own life that might be unnecessarily pushing her away from surveillance. For example, Olivia found a study about BRCA-positive women from different cultures. She found out that Scandinavian women rarely get prophylactic surgery, while the highest rate of prophylactic surgery is in the United States. For Olivia, this "hit a nerve" and made her realize that she needn't follow the American attitude of trying to fix or eliminate problems as easily as possible. She seeks her own approach that resembles other cultures' attitudes: "You can just live with sad news and deal with it . . . protect yourself, but not go to these extremes to fix everything."

Considerations about children and marriage weren't big factors in Olivia's decision. She's unsure whether she wants either and is focused on her career. In light of the BRCA diagnosis, her father has helped Olivia reframe her outlook from long-term to short-term planning. He acknowledges that "something bad is going to happen, more likely than not," whereas her mother's attitude is more characterized by denial. But it's okay that something bad will happen. Getting diagnosed with the BRCA mutation made Olivia feel that life is short and meant to be enjoyed, for the better. But it's also caused her to doubt whether she wants children.

> I do have this feeling right now that I know how I'm going to die. And it's weird to think that. And the only thing I think it's really changed about my future is now I'm thinking, I have to really want kids if I'm willing to subject them to potentially losing their mother at, like, in their late teens, or before they're fully grown, or having breast cancer with kids. And I think my decision to have kids, I'm less sure now than I was before . . . I don't feel like it's a good situation to be in, to feel like you have to question whether you want to have kids because you can't guarantee them as much . . . I feel sad.

Olivia has also turned to online communities for BRCA-positive mutation women for information and support, but is a critical reader. She thinks these websites and the women who use them are generally pro-surgery.

> The nature of the website is [pro-surgery] . . . I think that women who tend to post on websites . . . are more likely to have a personality that's more take-charge. Or, they identify more with BRCA. So then they tend to be more likely to, um, to take more extreme paths. I think it did affect me in the beginning, when I had less information. Now, but

I think that I've been able to formulate my own thoughts about it. But I did take about a week off the website, definitely, to think harder about what I felt.

What she read online affected her a lot more when she first got the BRCA test, before she was able to "formulate [her] own thoughts about it." Olivia continues to use the websites now that she has a better perspective on her BRCA-positive status and what she wants to do about it. The websites are useful for her because the extreme pro-surgery attitudes online balance out the lack of urgency of her family and friends who are not BRCA positive. Her loved ones simply haven't had her experience and don't relate to the enormity of dealing with being BRCA positive.

Olivia describes her surveillance decision as an empowering one that wasn't influenced by other people so much that the decision wasn't her own. She resents the attitude of women who are proactive about surgery and seem to judge those who choose surveillance. She feels that they chastise women who opt out of surgery for not acknowledging the importance of the BRCA mutation, a charge Olivia vehemently denies. If Olivia were to see herself in the future, she thinks that the only thing that could change her mind about having a prophylactic mastectomy would be to have children, which would make her feel "a stronger responsibility to . . . do everything in my power to stay alive." Right now, Olivia doesn't feel responsible to anyone but herself, and she isn't sure if she'll have kids in the next five years. By choosing surveillance, she is following a different but just as valid path to address her cancer risk.

Olivia's decision to choose surveillance came through a careful weighing of the medical statistical risk of developing cancer, as well as the social, individual, and psychological factors and influences in personal life. Good insurance coverage meant she didn't have to factor cost into her decision. As time goes on, I imagine that Olivia's outlook on career and family may change and alter her post–testing route. She has already hinted at how children would change her priorities. For now, though, Olivia is certain that surveillance is the right path for her as she faces her cancer risk.

With a lot of information and support both online and offline, Olivia felt empowered to "formulate my own thoughts about" choosing between surgery and surveillance. She takes in diverse opinions and remains in control of her own decision-making process, and is not pressured to obey one particular voice except her own. She sometimes wishes that she didn't know her

BRCA status, but overall she's glad she took the test. Being BRCA-positive mutation carrier, has become a part of her identity, but not in a terrible way: "kind of like something that's a part of you that's not going to define you."

Reluctant Gambler: June's Story

Sadly, not every woman is so confident in her decision to go with surveillance. We first met June in chapter 3 and saw her struggle over her family's disagreement with her decision to get tested for the BRCA mutation. June is in her early thirties, and has spent much of her late twenties and early thirties waiting for cancer to come. Having being diagnosed with Crohn's disease at a young age, June has long struggled with illness and been aware of her heightened cancer risk. She first suggested the BRCA test to her doctors in her early twenties.

> I came across a study that I read that, you know, people who have more flare ups have a higher chance of getting cancer, and stuff like that, of course, through the intestine. So because your entire, it's, it could affect your entire digestive tract, the inflammation. It was at my annual physical. When I went to a doctor and I brought the idea up . . . I was twenty, no more than. . . . Basically I say, "Do you think it's possible?" And the doctors say, "Yeah. It's possible, you know, because if you have relatives, and then plus given that you have other ailments that aren't very, a very pretty site in terms of like inflammation and stuff like that." . . . I waited, I waited. I didn't do it right away [laughing]. I didn't have the guts to find out.

Not until she was twenty-six did June really begin struggling with the fear of breast cancer. That's when she developed a breast lesion that did not heal and her doctor recommended the BRCA test. This recommendation was based also on the knowledge that June's great-grandmother had died of cancer, which she thinks was ovarian, and other relatives had died of various cancers. Her parents emigrated from China to the United States just after World War II and June has limited knowledge of her family's history of cancer.

When her BRCA test came back positive for the BRCA mutation, June felt that she wanted to have surgery right away. But when she told her parents about her BRCA status, they recommended she instead increase surveillance on her breasts and develop healthier eating habits. She notes:

I would have to say my family would not agree with me, how I feel, you know? It's like they don't believe in finding out. So they just believe in fate, you know? If they don't see anything is wrong, they're not going to do any protective measure in advance. But only when they're told that something is wrong, then they'll fix it. . . . They would not, never agree with, like what I wanted to do was have the surgery before the cancer attacked me. They don't agree with it. I'm on my own. They don't think that's necessary. They think, "What if it never happens?" . . . They would never agree to [surgery]. They don't think it's necessary to subject yourself to, you know, that kind of a treatment.

Let's just say I went in for my exam and they found a lump. I have cancer, right? Then, yes, [according to my family] of course I need to have the surgery to get rid of the cancer. But right now, I don't have cancer. I'm just carrying the gene. Maybe the gene will never happen. Maybe I'll live till I'm sixty before it happens. . . . For me, I don't agree with [my family].

June is the eldest of her siblings, and her younger sister thinks her surgical choice is "silly." June is generally very close to her family, so their feelings have a lot of impact. She doesn't feel "strong enough" to go against her family's basic philosophy, which she terms "fatalism." Only once she was diagnosed with cancer would her family support surgery; but that might not happen until she is sixty years old, or never. But for now she is following her family's push toward surveillance, despite her own wishes.

June and her family are conflicted about the best way to deal with her cancer risk in part because of her experience with Crohn's disease. This chronic illness put her in and out of hospitals and led to multiple surgeries throughout her life. She feels this experience has given her a different perspective from the rest of her family.

Everyone else in the family hasn't gotten put in such a predicament that I'm in, you know. . . . My family is more healthy than I am. They don't have the problems I go through, so they're inside a more sheltered society than I am. They're not going to be like me, be more alert and [doing] advanced planning . . . trying to find out all this stuff about myself.

Having dealt so much with medical issues in her life, June is not afraid of "getting the truth" and taking proactive measures for her health. Her family doesn't have that experience.

As far as other social support, June tells me she has no close friends, so she's received advice from only her parents and siblings. June is unmarried and does not have children, so she is trying to make the best decision for herself and her own health. She has felt extremely alone in the decision-making process and this loneliness has become an unwanted barrier to pursuing surgery.

> Down the road I would [get a mastectomy] but like I said, you know, I haven't, you know, had any opportunity. You know how I, my doctor has—she's married now, so you know, it's like she's got a supportive boyfriend and all that. So there's more encouragement, like, in her situation, whereas I'm in this situation that I'm all by myself. I don't have a boyfriend to encourage or a husband. And my family doesn't have—hold the same value I do. So, I feel like I'm like a loner, you know?

A big factor in her feeling "stuck," as she terms it, is the lack of social support that she needs to overcome her parents' negativity.

As June entered her thirties, she grew more concerned about cancer and more eager to take action to keep her body from becoming a "ticking time bomb." She has recently looked for that missing but crucial social support by visiting online support groups for BRCA-positive mutation women. She has connected especially with one woman who has had a prophylactic mastectomy; June notes: "I didn't even know that is possible to get support until I just, you know, came across meeting a person who is now my friend from a BRCA online support group." She's taking the first steps to get the support she needs.

Before getting that support, until recently June had looked to news stories and the media to make sense of her experience. The media influenced her thinking about what to do with her positive diagnosis, and she said,

> I heard what happened to Christina Applegate, the actress [who was diagnosed with breast cancer and the BRCA1 gene mutation and got a prophylactic double mastectomy], and that's when I started using the Internet website, Google, and looking into the possibility of surgery. I emailed her as a long shot, I didn't think she would answer me, but she did!

June also was strongly influenced by an episode of *Law and Order: Special Victims Unit* that begins with a girl killing her recently divorced father's new girlfriend.

And then when the police recover the body . . . [the] first person they link to her death is dad. And then of course they ask the dad, "Why did you divorce your wife?" The dad goes on to say: "Well I divorced my wife because she became pathetically crazy ever since she was diagnosed with the BRCA positive gene. She had the surgery without, without anyone's consent because she thinks she's going to die of cancer." That really . . . was like me, you know? Why of all things, why would they air such a show? That episode really set off a negative feeling about surgery, you know, what my intentions are for myself, you know? In a way that episode was trying to tell me, "You're not going to find a guy that will be okay with it."

This television episode added fuel to her fear of getting tested and taking further preventive action without her family's support. The media only sent her mixed messages about what to do.

The frightening story on *Law & Order: Special Victims Unit* also hit a nerve in June because of her fear of how a potential partner would respond these decisions.

So I'm not sure what the future is. I mean, do you see any possibility of myself finding my significant other, you know? I mean, I don't know how, if I did go about and have the surgery, do you think this person can accept me the way I am? It puts me in a lot of these, you know, "What ifs." . . . Twenty-six is like prime time, you know, to have, you know, a love life, you know [laughing]. It's like, well how to you explain to that other person you don't have any breasts? [laughing] How do you explain to someone that you cannot have children, you know?

Before ever knowing her BRCA status, she struggled to fit the ideal of the "petite Chinese girl" thanks to pressure from her own culture and her parents themselves. Her mother grew up in China and came from an upper-class Chinese family where women were supposed to be dutiful wives and mothers. If June got surgery, how could she attract a man if she doesn't fit a certain idea of what a woman should be? Removing her breasts would leave her looking different from most other women. And removing her ovaries would prevent her and a future partner from having any children of their own. Her parents have expressed their concern that breast surgery would harm June's chances at marriage because of the "slimmer chance [she has] of finding somebody."

June feels like she's waiting for cancer to come: "For me, I know that, you know, all these things about myself that I know what I'm expecting. So let's just say tomorrow I go to the doctor, I find out that I do have breast cancer, correct? It's not going to surprise me." She doesn't see surveillance as an empowering path but instead one where she is constantly struggling with her BRCA-positive mutation status. She compares her feelings to what she read in a book about the stages of dealing with death. June is currently in the stage of denial and bargaining with God. To reach the stage of acceptance, she would need to have surgery "to move on and get it over with." June is still struggling to find the affirmation she needs to make that surgical decision and hopes to be encouraged by a genetics counselor and overcome her parents' disapproval.

When speaking with June, I got the overwhelming impression that her post–testing BRCA experience has been disempowering. She had not actively sought information about her BRCA status up until recently and, more importantly, does not have the support she needs to have preventive surgery. Only recently has she found the support of an online contact, but that hardly seems enough to get her through the difficulty of preparing for surgery, undergoing the challenging procedure, and dealing with its potential effects on her health, self-image, and social life. She is sticking with surveillance for now, but pursuing the support she needs to choose surgery.

When Surveillance Leads to Surgery

June and Olivia's stories have at least one thing in common: surveillance is (usually) temporary. As I noted at the beginning of the chapter, surveillance and surgery are not two paths that are easy to separate and define. Women often choose surveillance at first but as time passes, and perhaps as they complete other life milestones such as having children or reaching a certain age, they move toward the surgical option. Both Olivia and June are currently undergoing surveillance for BRCA-related cancers, but June is clearly ready to change paths, and Olivia is open to removing her ovaries once she turns forty.

Reflecting on my interviews with women, it does seem that most, if not all, women have had or plan to have some kind of preventive surgery in their lifetime. One woman I interviewed had not yet had surgery but intended to. She said, "I don't want to get cancer. Like, that's the bottom line. So I'm planning to do the prophylactic mastectomy, um, certainly before I'm thirty." She sees surveillance as a path that would cause her too much anxiety and simply not an option to choose for the long term. Surgery is often framed as the only way for a BRCA-positive mutation woman to really, definitively address her risk.

Although surveillance and surgery seem to be opposite responses to a positive BRCA status, both choices can lead in the same direction. Women often choose surveillance at first, but, as time passes and, perhaps, as they complete other milestones such as having children or reaching a certain age, they move toward the surgical option.

It seems, in fact, that most if not all of the women I interviewed have had or plan to have some kind of preventive surgery. One woman intends to have surgery so as to take an "aggressive" approach to her BRCA-positive status—because avoiding cancer is her "bottom line." She sees surveillance as a path that would cause her too much anxiety. It's simply not an option she can choose. Surgery, in many of these narratives, is framed as the only way for a BRCA-positive woman to *really*, definitively address her risk.

So what about surgery as a means of addressing a woman's risk of hereditary breast and ovarian cancer? The next chapter explores the surgical option. It looks at the reasons women delay surgery, and why they don't. And, like this chapter, it presents case studies that provide insight into the ways surgery can be empowering and disempowering for women.

FIVE

The Surgical Fix

The whole thing was one long nightmare.

It's a pity and a shame. Not to mention a pain and an expense, you know . . . but it's, it's sad . . . I liked my body. I liked it, it's my own real piece of real estate, you know . . . I didn't want to have to do that to it . . . I'm still recovering.

I'm still recovering.

How can you not have regret?

Anne's story exemplifies how a surgical outcome can become disempowering when women get tested and find out "almost out of the blue" that they are positive because while a close relative tested positive for the BRCA-mutation gene, there is no other evidence of a family history of cancer. This left Anne ill-prepared to cope with the significance of her BRCA-positive mutation status, and unable to take the time to gather the social support among her family and friends to take control over her post–testing decisions. Although she has found support from her husband, describing him as "very, very, very supportive," her disempowerment stems from her feeling that she is entangled in larger medical and social trends disabling her from fully being in control of her body.

This time period to become ready, however long it may be, is crucial for a woman to assess her risk for cancer, or to accomplish important goals such as getting married or having a child. So as we saw in chapter 4, the line between the surveillance and surgery is not fixed. It's constantly shifting. Many women will eventually make both choices—surveillance and surgery—when it comes to their breasts and ovaries. Others pursue both choices simultaneously: they will monitor either their breasts or their ovaries for cancer while having preventive surgery to remove one of these body parts. In this chapter, we look at the surgical decisions that women make. What leads them to surgery? And who leads them? Why do some women delay the decision? What makes a woman's decision about surgery empowering, such as it was for Caroline, whom we learn about, or disempowering, as it was for Anne?

Most BRCA-positive women will eventually choose to have preventive surgery to remove their breasts, ovaries, or both. Prophylactic mastectomy takes many forms, including radical (complete removal), skin sparing, and nipple sparing. Mastectomies can be followed by different kinds of breast reconstruction including implants, using a woman's own tissue to reform the breasts, and tattooing an areola and nipple. In order to reduce her risk of ovarian cancer, a woman can have an oophorectomy (remove her ovaries) and sometimes also a hysterectomy (completely remove her uterus). An oophorectomy can also reduce a woman's risk of breast cancer because ovaries secrete hormones that help cancerous cells grow elsewhere in the body. In this book, I generalize women's surgical options into the basic two: mastectomy and oophorectomy. I explain this in more detail when it's important to a woman's story.

For women who choose surgery, surveillance simply is not enough. They don't want to live with cancer or with their fear of cancer. In some women's lives, cancer is more like the elephant in the room—and it's not addressed. But for most, choosing surveillance alone is the epitome of waiting for cancer to come and is not how they want to live. Several women describe surveillance as a game of Russian roulette: you're playing a waiting game, never knowing when that gun pointed at your head will fire and you'll be diagnosed with cancer.

BRCA-positive mutation women see surgery as the most proactive and empowering way to face their risk of hereditary breast and ovarian cancer. Preventive surgery is perceived to stop the threat of cancer from overtaking their lives. There is the strong belief that it stops cancer before it can come. Women strongly believe that having surgery is the only way to take control of their lives and combat what would otherwise be their genetic destiny. What women are less likely to mention, though, is that preventive surgery does not entirely prevent the development of cancer—but it may greatly reduce the risk.

An important factor in a woman's decision about preventive surgery is how she calculates her personal risk of developing cancer. As we saw in chapter 4, many women equate a BRCA-positive mutation result with the inevitability of cancer such that the gap between risk and getting cancer becomes negligible. Many more evaluate their risk to be as high as 90 percent based on information provided by Myriad Corporation and their health-care providers. As one woman explains:

> [My doctor said] "Your chance of getting another breast cancer is, like, you know, 74 percent or 67 percent." It was some high number. . . . And I'm thinking, you know, I wouldn't get on a plane if they told me there's a 67 percent chance this plane's going down [laughs]. . . . And that's the way I think about it, you know. If they told me that, I would never get on that plane. . . . So I thought, I'm gonna have to do a double mastectomy now, 'cause I'm not doing chemo again. I cannot—I just couldn't do it.

This woman feels that preventive surgery will ensure that she never has to have chemotherapy again. But there is still a risk of developing breast or ovarian cancer after surgery because some tissue is always left behind. Nonetheless, most women consider surgery worth it because it does decrease the risk of cancer, and, sometimes, it feels as if surgery will eliminate this risk altogether.

What Kind of Surgery and When?

Many things affect whether and when a woman chooses surgery. Age and marital status both play a role, but most important are a woman's family history of cancer, whether she has children, and the influence of health-care providers and other women she meets through online support groups.

Overall, older women are more likely to have surgery. The average of age of the women I surveyed who had surgery was forty-one, and the average age of those who did not have surgery was thirty-five. A woman's marital and motherhood status also affects the surgical decision. Of the women who had surgery, over half had at least one child, and over 70 percent were married. In comparison, only 36 percent of women who elected surveillance were mothers and half were married. Women who already have children are more likely to remove their ovaries, which they no longer "need." We met Stephanie in chapter 2 and heard her describe the importance of already having children to electing surgery. When I spoke with Stephanie, she had already had a mastectomy and was soon going to have an oophorectomy. She said:

I talked to my husband about it a lot in the last couple months and, frankly we know we're done with kids. We've had four pregnancies, two miscarriages, two kids. You know, the whole thing is very stressful. We're very happy with our two girls. They're happy, they're healthy, they're beautiful, they're smart. We're done. Um, that aside, I have tons of issues with my ovaries. My ovulation kills me every month. My periods hurt. I got to the point where I'm like, "Why wait? I'm thirty one, why wait four more years?"

We're seeing the opposite effect of age and life status to what we saw in chapter 4. Once women accomplish certain life milestones and get older, they become ready to move from surveillance to surgery.

Women also choose surgery to ensure they will remain in their children's lives in the future. One woman said she is having surgery for her daughter's sake: "She needs me and I need to be here for her." Another explains, "I would never want my family to go through all this." Yet another says, "If one of us [my husband or I] passed away, we would be devastated, but you could go on with your life. But with kids, if we both go down, it was kind of Armageddon." When a woman has children, waiting for cancer to come is no longer an option. Women also feel that, by having preventive surgery, they are being good role models for their children, who might also have the BRCA mutation. One woman notes that she tried to keep a very optimistic attitude throughout her surgery for the sake of her daughter, who is also BRCA positive: "Everything I did I was thinking about my daughter." Another woman actually planned to have a mastectomy before having children in order to "forego the breastfeeding to be healthy for . . . [them] and to . . . be able to care for them without trying to recover from a surgery."

Whether a woman has the BRCA1 or BRCA2 gene mutation affects her likelihood of choosing preventive surgery. A woman with the BRCA1 gene mutation has a 60–90 percent risk of developing breast cancer in her life (based on a life expectancy of eighty-five years). A woman with the BRCA2 gene mutation has a lifetime risk is between 30–85 percent. Women with the BRCA1 gene also have a higher risk of developing ovarian cancer than do women who are BRCA2 positive—about a 55 percent lifetime risk compared to about a 25 percent risk. Unsurprisingly, more women diagnosed with the BRCA1 gene mutation elect preventive surgery. Because the risk of ovarian cancer is lower than the risk of breast cancer for both BRCA-positive groups, oophorectomy is less common than mastectomy. BRCA-positive women feel more leeway in deciding when and if they should get their ovaries removed, especially when there is no history of ovarian cancer in their families.

It's important to note that even BRCA1 and BRCA2 risk assessments are generalizations. While the genetic test is designed to look for both mutations, they also have many subtypes. A woman's risk for certain cancers varies based not only on the general categorization into either BRCA1 or BRCA2 but also on the subtype of genetic mutation diagnosed, when possible. Not all subtypes of the mutations have been identified. Women who are told that they have a rare variant of the BRCA1 or BRCA2 gene mutation may find it hard to calculate their risk because its unknown how aggressive that variant is. Some women use online forums to find others with their particular variant and to see how these other women have responded to the diagnosis.

A woman's health-care provider is evidently one of the first places she will get and seek advice about surgery. These experts are generally in the room when women decide to get tested, receive their results, and first start contemplating post–testing decisions. Some women change health-care providers frequently to find the best match, while others develop close relationships with their providers over time. Regardless however, a woman's doctors, counselors, and other providers are an important front-line source of advice when it comes to choosing preventive surgery. Many encourage BRCA-positive mutation women to have surgery. Some even frame cancer as inevitable, and preventive surgery as the right answer to address their hereditary cancer risk. Later we hear Liz's story. One of her doctors told her: "You have to have a mastectomy." Another woman's doctor was entirely blunt in promoting surgery, saying, "You will not turn forty with your ovaries if I am your doctor."

Within their families, many women see themselves as the BRCA-positive mutation pioneers of their families if they are the first to get tested, especially if they are the first to elect preventive surgery. These women are setting the bar for their relatives and often become a source of information, guidance, and support for others to choose surgery as well. One of the women I spoke with described herself and her sister, the only members of their extended family to get prophylactic mastectomies, as "the pioneers of leading this new charge of breaking the curse."

The Mother's Cancer Clock in Surgical Decision Making

A significant theme throughout many of women's stories was how they based their own choices for preventative surgery or surveillance by their memories and experiences with their mothers' struggles with cancer. Just as Christina and Kelsey did in chapter 3 when they were deciding whether to get tested, or like Susan calculating her own risk of cancer based upon her mother's and oldest sister's experiences, a woman's surgical decision also incorporates her own family's history of cancer. A woman's mother's experience is especially important; a woman who lost her mother to breast cancer tends to have surgery more quickly after a BRCA-positive mutation diagnosis than a woman who has not. Research on women's experience with genetic testing has noted the importance of social networks—the people they know—in women's post–testing decision making, especially with regard to women's firsthand experiences of dealing with cancer in their families (Chalmers and Thomson 1996; D'Agincourt-Canning and Baird 2006; Hallowell et al. 2001; Lee 2010; Mellon et al. 2009).

Surgery is more likely for a woman who has multiple family members that have been diagnosed with cancer or has lost a close relative to cancer. Living with cancer in her family can heighten a woman's fear that cancer is inevitable. This feeling came across in many of the stories of the women I interviewed. As they spoke about their memories of their families' battles with cancer, they expressed similar feelings of inevitability and the fear of waiting for cancer to come. As one woman from a family with a strong cancer history said about getting her BRCA-positive mutation diagnosis, "It was pretty clear to me . . . that I should have had breast cancer." Another, whose mother and aunt are cancer survivors, notes, "One day it's my turn. I'm going to have cancer." A third woman, whose mother survived breast cancer, described her feelings after getting the BRCA-positive news: "Every day was full of pain and terror. It's a matter of when I get cancer, not if I get cancer."

This heightened fear and this sense of the inevitable leads many women to preventive surgery, such as one woman whose mother and aunt died of breast cancer. She explained to me that she thought of her mother when she decided to get a mastectomy, noting, "I was probably thinking about [my mother] . . . how young she was when she got cancer . . . how I was now older than she was when she got it." One woman whose mother died of breast cancer when she was thirteen explains how this set her on the course of being extremely careful about her preventative care: "It began there . . . when, you know, your mother passes away of such a disease, when you get older, you know, very precautious about it. Very cautious about it . . . [I] always went for my, my tests, always went for breast exams." She ended up having a double mastectomy and a hysterectomy. Another woman based her surgical decisions entirely on her family history—specifically her mother's and her grandmothers' deaths from breast cancer—rather than on medical advice. She wasn't testing for the BRCA mutation gene, but explained to me that throughout her extensively thought-out decision making, she ultimately came to one conclusion:

> Me having the surgery . . . it's like, "Okay, well that's something that's [I] felt [I] needed to do." . . . I put it in my head that even if I got tested and I was negative that I would still do it just because there's so many things we don't know about our genes and, um, I just felt like I was at high risk no matter what.

Thus it was her family history that guided her as she decided the best course of action for preventing cancer: a double mastectomy.

Family narratives of hereditary cancer for many women will guide their medical decision making, perhaps even more so than medical recommendations or statistics on illness and survival (Babb et al 2002; Erblich, Bovbjerg, and Valdimarsdottir 2000; Kenen, Arden-Hones, and Eeles 2003; Werner-Lin 2007). This was certainly true in the stories of the women I spoke with. My respondents use their family history, and specifically their mother's timelines as a guide for their own decision making. For many women, such as Jennifer—whom we met in chapter 2, and whose mother died from breast cancer when Jennifer was only six months old—the loss of a mother, grandmother, sister, or aunt will frame their own surgical decision making for the rest of their lives, as these women become part of the family narrative. For some women then, surgery allows women to challenge their cancer history, and to exert control over how the narrative will continue; hopefully toward a happier conclusion for the family legacy than they remember.

"A Community of Women": Finding Support Online

Sometimes a woman doesn't find enough—or any—support from her family or health-care providers. She may need to hear from another woman who has gone through the same things she has—and sometimes it seems like no one else has. Online support groups often help fill that gap. Reading other women's stories and sometimes meeting other BRCA-positive mutation women in person can help women throughout the BRCA process. Although these groups aim to be open to many ideas and the different decisions women make, women tend to see online support groups for BRCA-positive women as pro-surgery. We heard Olivia's story in chapter 4, so we know she was hesitant to rely too much on websites geared toward BRCA-positive women. She describes reading many stories of women who have had surgery and feels as though the websites are harboring a "culture of fear . . . that you're waiting to have the ball drop."

Even if they're biased, these groups are invaluable sources of support for many women. Some women may even feel unable to face their risk without leaning on others going through similar experiences. When no one in a woman's family or circle of friends has been diagnosed as BRCA positive and no one has had to make the difficult decisions that come with it, such as whether to have children, she can feel lost and alone. Who can help? Online support groups provide that important connection to a seemingly endless number of women going through the BRCA experience. A woman may just read message boards, add comments or her own story, e-mail and chat with other women, or go so far as to bridge her online and off-line lives by meeting up with women she met online.

When most women in the United States have not taken the BRCA test, entering the world of online support groups can make a woman realize she is not alone. These communities were very important to Jessica. They did not necessarily help her make a decision about surgery, but they did comfort her as she went through her own post–testing decision-making process. They made her feel like she "just wasn't so alone." Her own family members didn't understand why she would make such a drastic choice as preventive surgery. She notes, "These people on that website are in my shoes . . . regardless of their decision, they all know the stress of it all." While Jessica relied on websites for general support rather than for help with her decision, for others, online support groups can be critical in their choice to have preventive surgery. Such is the case for Emily.

Finding Online Support: Emily's Story

Emily first went online to research information about her surgery. She has a personal strategy for dealing with online information.

> I've just been doing a lot of information gathering on the web and trying to form, sort of, gather the facts and get them straight in my head, and then form sort of tentative, um, tentative plans, or tentative ideas about the best way to move forward. And sort of see what the doctors say. And often, doctors will say something that I think, "This doesn't

quite sound right to me." So then I go back to the web and I do a little more. In fact, I have actually—I went on the message board at one point, and said, "Okay, guys, here's what a doctor told me. Is this consistent with what all of your doctors have told you?" And I got back a lot of different responses with a variety of perspectives. And so, I guess I do, probably, gosh. I've done a lot on the web. It's probably eighty or eighty-five percent fact finding that way. And usually by the time I get to the doctors, I'm kind of asking the really detailed, nitty-gritty questions because I've already kind of figured out the more basic stuff.

For this reason, Emily has found online BRCA-related resources, particularly the FORCE (Facing Our Risk of Cancer Empowered) website, which deals specifically with women who have the BRCA mutation, "indispensable" to her post–testing life and decision-making.

Going online ended up also providing Emily the support of women in similar situations. Message boards are a place for dialogue with and among "a community of women."

> They're the only people on Earth who are just like you. And you get a variety of perspectives of, you know, people ask questions about, you know, "What kind of surgery should I have?" Or "I'm having these symptoms, what could that mean?" It's just really useful. And then, even a before and after page where you can see photos of women before and after their mastectomies. . . . So it's really, I have found this website absolutely, just indispensable. And I cannot imagine what women did before this website came into being.

This community of women was also a sounding board for Emily's concerns and a source of feedback on medical advice, especially when she felt uncertain about that advice or received conflicting opinions.

As well as providing a connection to other BRCA-positive mutation women, the FORCE website features a before and after photo gallery of women who have had mastectomies. Emily points to this gallery as important in two different ways for women who are considering or preparing for preventive surgery: they can get a sense of what to expect, and they understand that they are not alone when they see that other women have been through surgery. As important is that, although these women may not look "perfect," they still "look pretty good" and, as many BRCA-positive women believe, will not get cancer.

Going online really did help Emily decide on which treatment was best for her. Her doctor recommended that she get a certain type of post–mastectomy reconstruction with implants. However, Emily made a different choice.

> Long story short, after hours and hours and hours and hours . . . on the web, ordering books that I learned about on the web, reading those books, etc. . . . I realized I don't want implants. I want another type of reconstruction. . . . Without the Internet, I never would have come to that. I just would have said, "Well, gee, you're the doctor, you know best."

Online, Emily discovered reconstructive options that her doctor hadn't mentioned. Without this information, she would have been less able to decide for herself what type of surgery she wanted, and she would have deferred to her doctor's recommendation.

Although Emily praises and supports online resources and communities for BRCA-positive women such as FORCE, she is careful to add a warning. Women who use the Internet to gather information and facts, like she did, need to read carefully. A woman should be especially cautious when reading message boards, Emily believes. "You don't know who is making that post, and you don't know anything about that person, and you don't know whether they really know what they're talking about or not." It is a mistake to "just believe" information that may be posted on message boards and, in general, information taken from the Internet should be taken "with a grain of salt."

Overall, though, Emily views the Internet as an extraordinarily helpful and supportive tool that helps BRCA-positive mutation women find information, individual opinions, and personal stories. She "cannot imagine what women did before [the FORCE] website came into being." Emily has used FORCE and other online resources as central tools to help her to figure out how to handle her BRCA-positive diagnosis in a way that is best for her. Pairing her doctors' recommendations with facts found online allows Emily to access a wide range of options. In the end, she finds the Internet truly indispensable because it allows her to find the post–diagnosis path that's most comfortable for her.

Delaying Surgery

As we saw in chapters 3 and 4, many women who put off getting tested, and when they are tested then choose to practice surveillance and delay preventative surgery, feel empowered by their medical decisions because they perceive these option as a way to buy time in order to accomplish other goals in their lives such as finishing their degree, getting married, having children, and so on.

There is a sense among women who elect surgery that the time was ripe for them to move forward. Once they decide to do so, they then get tested and schedule surgery very quickly. As one women told me "what's the sense in my getting tested if I am not ready to get surgery?" For these women, to get tested is to learn something they already knew years before—that they were already BRCA positive, such as in Jennifer's story. The phrase I heard among women who were empowered by their surgical decision was, "I already knew, but I didn't want to know." One woman in the study in fact said that she was ready to get surgery and that she really didn't need to get tested before her surgical decision, because she knew already that she was BRCA positive and didn't need a test result to tell her.

Waiting to be tested when you feel ready, then becomes an important empowerment tool that women utilize to take control over their lives, allowing them to keep cancer in abeyance, until they feel ready to be tested. Being ready encompasses a whole range of important life issues. It is this process of getting ready, which for some in my study took many decades, but once they felt ready, all things seemed to fall into place. As one woman who had surgery described to me, after she waited almost two decades to be tested, her feeling of being ready was the" perfect storm", where all things in her life came together to enable her to move forward with testing, while she already knew that she would have surgery immediately afterwards.

As we have seen, BRCA-positive women decide to get surgery at different times after being diagnosed. While some women know exactly what they plan to do before ever getting tested, others find the positive result a shock and must take time to weigh their options before making any decisions. Many women will start with surveillance but move to the surgical category. One woman describes surveillance as "just a stop gap until you're ready to get" surgery. All women must answer the same basic questions. What kind of surgery do I want? Do I need to address my risk for breast or ovarian cancer right now—or both? Are there other things in my life, like having children, which need to happen before I can get surgery? Am I okay with losing my breasts?

With so many questions to ask themselves, many women delay surgery until they are comfortable with the answers. In contrast, some women get tested and jump into surgery immediately once they discover they are BRCA positive. Several of the women I spoke with had a preventive mastectomy within just a few months of receiving their test results, scheduling the surgery the same day if not before. Some women also decide quickly to have an oophorectomy or hysterectomy; one woman said she couldn't "get the ovaries out fast enough." They're not waiting for cancer to come.

Different circumstances cause women to delay either or both of their surgeries. One research study defined the right time for BRCA-positive women to have preventive surgery to be determined by several things, including having time to think about the decision, fitting the surgery into current and future life plans, and feeling that genetic and medical knowledge is advanced enough to make surgery a viable and effective option (Howard et al. 2010). Choosing surgery and choosing BRCA testing actually involve similar processes. Women must also be ready for surgery.

This was the case for both Caroline and Kelsey, two women I talk more about later on in this chapter. Caroline knew immediately that she would have preventative surgery after getting tested for BRCA because, as she explained to me, "part of the reason I didn't want to get tested very young is because I didn't think that I was ready to have that surgery, and I knew that if I had the gene that's exactly what I would do." So Caroline waited to get tested and have an oophorectomy and mastectomy until she was mentally ready. And ready for Caroline meant her kids being older, so she has more time and energy to devote to her health and well being during the surgery. Caroline also felt ready after discussing the surgery with her cousin, and after feeling that she needed to take action before she reaches the age that her relatives got cancer. Kelsey has similar feelings. While she is determined to have preventative surgery done, when I interviewed her, Kelsey was still in the surveillance phase, not quite yet ready to have the surgery done.

The women who delay getting an oophorectomy or hysterectomy feel they have time to wait on their ovaries—and they want to have a family first. But women are torn when they have an increased risk for ovarian cancer not only because of their BRCA-positive diagnosis but also because the disease runs in the family. On the one hand, their doctors tell them they can wait. The age they should wait for (based on the recommendations of health-care providers) seems to vary, tending to range from thirty to forty. Regardless of the advice from their doctors, some women turn to their families' cancer history for guidance.

Rachel said, "I couldn't get my surgery scheduled fast enough," after getting the BRCA test. A decade earlier, her mother died of ovarian cancer. Her mother's first cousin died of the disease shortly thereafter. Rachel knew she wanted to be tested for a long time, but doctors did not allow her to for several years. When she finally switched doctors, got the test, and tested positive, she was shocked. She scheduled surgery immediately. Rachel was especially worried because she was approaching the age when her first cousin had died. When reflecting on other women's experiences, she realizes the surgical decision is probably easier to make when you witness family members die of cancer.

Rachel was also comfortable with the surgery because she had an eighteen-year-old son and knew she and her husband were not going to have more children. This "took out some stress" because she didn't have to decide between having children and having surgery. Her decision would have been much more difficult at a different time in her life. If she were single, she wouldn't have had her family's support when she had her surgery. And at the time of her surgery, her son was old enough to take care of himself. She remains positive about the oophorectomy, saying that surgery "beats dying" and leaving her son without a parent.

Finances did not impact Rachel's decision but can be an important part of a woman's decision. Some women, for example, get surgery because their insurance companies won't cover surveillance measures. Others wait until they have saved enough money to afford preventive surgery and time off work for recovery.

The Surgical Fix: Empowering and Disempowering

A woman chooses preventive surgery to take control of her fate. But the rate at which women increasingly elect preventive surgery—more so than most other countries—is troubling for many. Research studies on how women decide between treatment options suggests that women tend to inflate their risk in ways that often lead them to inappropriate choices, including risky preventive surgeries such as preventive mastectomies or oophorectomies (Heshka et al. 2008; Sivell et al. 2008). There is often a disconnect in whether surgery is considered a good choice between researchers and women themselves.

Assessing women's surgical judgment as good or bad from a health-care provider's point of view, however, is often to negatively judge women's surgical choices, without really listening to the experiences and concerns that drive their medical decision making. If medical personnel seek to both be part of, and to positively influence, this process, it is imperative that they begin this understanding with women's lived realities. This is especially true regarding how women come to perceive the process and the outcome of their medical decisions, and the extent to which they feel empowered while doing so.

These feelings of empowerment or disempowerment depend on women's abilities to feel that they can take hold of and shape their lives. Many women find their surgeries inherently empowering because they strongly believe that their choice to get surgery will lead to eliminating the threat of cancer. As one woman notes, "I really wanted to do something, to take control." Others, too, describe surgery as giving them the power to prevent death by cancer. When women are tired of waiting for cancer to come, surgery is the best option to end the wait. In reality, though, surgery might not be as empowering for a woman as she hoped. The next two women's stories look at the different factors in a woman's life that can make her empowered and disempowered by choosing surgery.

"There Was No Question": Caroline's Story

Soon after learning her BRCA-positive mutation status, Caroline decided to get preventive surgery to reduce her risk of both ovarian and breast cancer. When we spoke, she was thirty-six and married with two children. Her doctor recommended the BRCA test because of her extensive family history of breast, ovarian, and pancreatic cancer. She didn't get tested immediately, however, but waited until her children were older and she was around the age that other family members had been diagnosed with cancer. It wasn't until then that she felt more prepared to deal with the meaning of a BRCA-positive mutation test. What finally pushed her over the edge was her cousin's BRCA-positive mutation test result.

Based on her family's history of cancer, Caroline always knew she'd have to deal with it herself, because: "I just knew I had the gene mutation." One factor enabling her to take the test was being prepared for next steps. Caroline saw herself as having a choice between cancer and surgery, and that was not a difficult decision for her to make.

> [After getting tested in September], I had an oophorectomy in November, and just in March I had a prophylactic mastectomy. I did a lot of reading on [the FORCE website], and, you know, I had seen, my cousin did, as soon as she had her test, did the same thing. And I saw her go through her surgeries. And I guess I kind of felt like I knew

that I was going to expect, you know what I mean? Like I knew what was going to happen. And honestly, this is going to sound crazy, but I thought it was more painful giving birth.

Caroline describes her surgeries as "literally a breeze"—she had no trouble with the surgeries themselves or the recovery process. She had support from her husband, from the cousin who had already had surgery, and from her sister, who planned her own surgeries with Caroline and had both those surgeries on the same dates. Caroline's surgeries were relatively easy because she saw, through the FORCE message boards, "that there [were] other people dealing with the same stuff."

Most important in making Caroline's experience an empowering one is her own confidence in preventive surgery being her own decision, and the right one. As she says, "I knew that if I had the gene [preventive surgery is] exactly what I would do." She trusted the doctors who performed the surgery and felt supported by women going through similar experiences.

> I know this sounds crazy, but we were like, okay, it's like a ticking time bomb. Get them off, you know. [On FORCE] it was nice to see that there were other people dealing with the same stuff. The fact that I could prevent, or, you know, attempt to prevent, reduce my risk significantly, was huge. I don't know why people have such bad experiences. I don't know if that's because they weren't ready, if their doctors maybe weren't right for them, I'm not sure. I knew what I was going to do was going to be good for me in the end, and I had no negative feeling about it.

Her experience was positive because she owned her choice: "I did it for the right reason, for myself. I was ready to do it." This personal sentiment was echoed in Kelsey's story, who told me that preventative surgery was certainly the choice for her. While Kelsey is taking some time with surveillance before actually getting her surgery, she says:

> There's nothing I can do about having this gene, but there's a lot I can do about making it a better situation. And you know, I—I don't think that people would really understand, like, the choice to do the mastectomy. Um, but, you know, for me at this point, it's a no-brainer. Just, it just comes down to that I don't want to get cancer.

Kelsey shares Caroline's feelings about surgery that it is the best course of action to survive. Kelsey was adamant that "I'm not going to get cancer," and she will ensure this by preventative means. Caroline similarly felt that after verifying that she is BRCA positive that "there was no question what I was going to do."

Because this was such a determined personal decision, Caroline had a positive post–surgical experience. She says, "My clothes look good, I feel good, I'm, you know, back to the gym, back to working out. I feel really good." Caroline describes herself as a "positive person" and says:

> I'm ready to move on and focus on what's important: my family, my kids, my students . . . I'm not that person to dwell on the situation. If there's a problem, I would discuss it and move on, you know what I mean? And I think that's how I'm looking at this. Okay, there's an issue, let's address it, and I'm ready to move on. It's just a small portion of who I am, you know what I mean? It's not something that I'm going to dwell on. I think that can really bring you down.

Having addressed the "issue" of being BRCA-positive mutation carrier, Caroline can now leave it behind. Being BRCA positive no longer defines her experience or weighs on her regularly.

Surgery is empowering for Caroline for a number of reasons. As we saw, the most important is her confidence that she made her own decision in her own time. Seeing the devastation of cancer firsthand among her relatives made Caroline strongly believe that her decision was right; preventive surgery was the positive step she needed to take to avoid that fate. Like many women, she planned before being tested to have preventive surgery if she were a BRCA-positive mutation carrier. Caroline also had support for her decision from close family members.

Women often experience being ready for testing and preventive surgery as intertwined, and they move forward with both at the same time. The BRCA test only tells Caroline and other women something they "already knew" long before: they are at a high risk for cancer. One of the women I interviewed was so compelled by her family history that she decided to get preventive surgery without even getting tested. She didn't need the positive result to know her risk. And surgery can often be empowering. Caroline says, "I would do it all over again in a second."

Unfortunately, not all women are empowered by having prophylactic surgery. The next story shows how getting your BRCA-positive mutation results before you are ready can leave you ill-prepared to cope with the significance of the result. Women need time to get social support for their decisions, whether from family, friends, or other sources. Being rushed into any decision without that support can leave women unhappy about their decisions.

"I Went in Blind": Liz's Story

Because her mother died of breast cancer, Liz began practicing surveillance at age twenty-nine, and she chose to have the BRCA test as soon as her physician recommended it to her. She always sought to be proactive about her cancer risk, and she "just knew" her BRCA results would come back positive, even before she saw them. After taking the test, Liz immediately agreed to continue regular screening, as her geneticist recommended. She felt surveillance was the right path for her.

> I walk in [to get my results] and they're all looking at me and I could tell from their faces that I was positive, so that—And then I walk in with the counselor, and was, "Just say it!" And she said it. And, "How do you feel?" And I said, "Okay. I wanna go shopping." She, we met two weeks ago, and I said this to her, and she cracked up laughing 'cause she said she had never had anyone say that to her. It was like, okay, you confirmed what I already knew, so now I wanna move on with my life.

Getting the BRCA test didn't really change Liz's life but reinforced her need for screening.

However, another medical professional soon told Liz outright that this was the wrong choice—that mammography and MRIs alone were "not enough" to prevent cancer.

> [The doctor] said, "No, it's not enough." . . . She told me, you have to have a mastectomy. . . . And that one sentence did it for me. By the time I came in, from Monday to Friday, with my husband, at her office, and I said to her, get all the papers [to have surgery] around, and whatever she wants to tell me. . . . Let's do it.

Such a forceful, direct statement made Liz feel as though her options were either to have preventive surgery and avoid cancer or to continue with surveillance and inevitably develop cancer. She did not like this advice but felt she had no one else to turn to for an alternative perspective. She notes, "I had no information. I went in blind . . . I had my doctor and their nurses, and everybody was great, but that's all." With no one to balance her doctor's extreme perspective, she came to a stark conclusion: "If I continue with surveillance, I guess I die."

Liz thus elected to have a preventive double mastectomy and a hysterectomy. Although her doctor's words gave her the biggest push toward surgery, Liz was also influenced by her mother's death from breast cancer and her trust in the breast surgeon, whom she had seen for ten years prior to the prophylactic surgeries. These two factors show that Liz's decision was not entirely forced upon her. Nevertheless, her choice to have surgery resulted in part from the powerful advice of medical professionals who made her feel she needed to have surgery or would die, a false ultimatum.

Liz's experience is disempowering not only because of the circumstances leading up to the surgeries but also because she is uncertain about her decision when she reflects on it. Some research suggests that women who elect surgery or surveillance but are uncertain about the decision may experience higher levels of anxiety over their choice of treatment, whichever choice they make, than women who are confident in their treatment choice (Litton et al. 2009). Making a sudden change from surveillance to surgery left Liz fraught with uncertainty.

But Liz cannot go back to a time prior to her surgical procedure, so she is in the process of moving forward. She hopes to gain empowerment from her surgical decision by claiming this decision as her own and seeing it as the best route to eradicating her cancer risk. She ultimately came to terms with the decision and says she would do it again. Fortunately, Liz's experience with the surgeries themselves was positive, because she accepts her new body and had a normal recovery period. She feels that preventive surgery was the right decision for her health and has the support of her husband, who is unconditionally helpful and "left it totally up to [her]." Liz's decisions were neither dictated nor questioned by her loved ones, and, despite the undue influence of her doctor, in this way, they were her own.

Looking Back: Surgery or Surveillance?

We've heard many women's stories over the past two chapters. Women who chose surgery or surveillance or both; women who easily made these decisions or struggled for some time. At least one thing is clear: after getting their BRCA-positive mutation result, women do not follow a traditionally "rational" medical model of statistical risk assessment. They don't take for granted the statistical data provided by their genetics counselors or doctors. Each woman reframes her risk to reflect a broader nexus of decision-making that includes her family history and the amount of support and information available to her through her social network of family, friends, and, increasingly, online relationships. How a woman calculates her risk directly affects her post–testing medical decisions.

Women who elect to have preventive surgery soon after getting their positive mutation result have often directly experienced a close family member dying of cancer. Their experiences tend to differ from those of the women we met in chapter 4, who elect surveillance and, most often, have not seen a mother, sister, brother, or child die from cancer. As we also saw in chapter 4, women who elect surveillance, and who are, on average, young, feel they still have time on their side as the continue to negotiate their BRCA-positive mutation status.

Whether they choose surveillance or surgery, women use the cancer history of their families, especially the age at which relatives were diagnosed (if known), to help them calculate their own cancer risk or how much time they may have before cancer strikes. Women who elect preventive surgery tend to believe that surgery is the only way to "fix" things and, often, that it can eliminate the threat of cancer. This view comes from a larger idea of genetic determinism where getting a BRCA-positive mutation result means inevitably getting cancer. As one woman said, she is waiting for "not if, but when cancer comes." Genetic testing and surgery provide BRCA-positive women with a pathway they feel will change their genetic destiny and end what one respondent calls the "BRCA curse."

Yes, some women who choose surveillance also link a BRCA-positive mutation diagnosis with getting cancer. But they don't express the same sense of urgency regarding the need for surgery. Instead, they feel they can buy time before they get cancer. Women currently undergoing surveillance and those who once practiced it but eventually chose surgery often liken surveillance to a holding pattern. In fact, many who have chosen one surgery or another are still holding—waiting to have that other surgery. They continue surveillance for ovarian cancer, for example, and wait to get their ovaries removed at a later date because they want more children or hope to avoid the onset of early menopause. Others wait because they're not ready for surgery. Perhaps they want to get married or launch their careers first. Of course, there are some exceptions. For example, young unmarried women without children may choose surgery to free themselves up and get on with their lives or to avoid the fate of a close relative who died of cancer at a young age.

Although some women experience very difficult surgeries and reconstruction that leaves them with negative feelings about their bodies, preventive surgery is empowering for most women. Why? By and large, women who have surgery have an unwavering belief in the power of preventive surgery to eradicate their risk and take away their fear of getting cancer. The minority of women who are disempowered by surgery do not claim the decision as their own and they do not feel they were ready to make that decision. Often, they rely heavily on the advice of their doctors, electing preventive surgery despite their own reservations.

What have we learned? In the end, a woman can be empowered regardless of her treatment choice as long as she takes control of the decision-making process. Women who feel empowered by their treatment decisions often seek information from alternative, nonmedical sources—from family and friends and websites written by women with similar experiences. They consider all these factors as they decide. They discuss options with medical providers, ask questions, and make their own choices, sometimes in the face of opposition from loved ones or from medical professionals who disagree with their decision.

By listening carefully to women's experiences, we have uncovered the ways in which women encounter dominant medical beliefs and treatment systems. Traditional ways of looking at women's decisions assume they will follow a rational decision-making process once a medical professional informs them of their genetic risk. These models do not begin to capture the variety and depth of the decision-making processes that BRCA-positive mutation women actually engage in.

If we want to maximize cancer prevention strategies for BRCA-positive mutation women, it is critical for care providers such as oncologists and genetic counselors to understand decision-making from the perspective of BRCA-positive mutation women. These health-care professionals must understand which factors within the medical environment serve to empower or disempower these women as they decide which choice is best for them. We will see more evidence for this in the next chapters when we look at the broader impact of a positive BRCA diagnosis on women's lived experiences.

SIX

Finding a New Normal

After surgery, my breasts were a little smaller than they were before. I had very large breasts before. I always kind of had a hard time wearing tank tops and other things just because I didn't want to look, you know, too over the top or anything. So I went about a size smaller when I got my surgery, which has been nice. And it's also been nice, you know, I don't have to wear a bra anymore, which is awesome. So there's a couple perks to having breast surgery.

I'm definitely used to these breasts. No one can make it as good as God can. And they're definitely not as great as my old ones. And I definitely still miss them and wish I could feel things again. But when I look at them, they're fine. And you know, I have scars, and it's fine. And when I wear clothes, you know, you can't even tell most of the time. Whenever I'm wearing clothes it's fine. I'm getting used to them.

I'm doing a lot better than I was six months ago. It's the new normal you know? I, I've been through a lot. I obviously have grown a lot and gotten a lot stronger as a person through all this. I don't sweat the small stuff. I've had to come to peace with myself and kind of what I've been through, I mean, it's tough and I'm still fragile and I still get upset sometimes when like a couple weeks ago, I was at a swimming party with a bunch of my friends, and walked outside and my nipple was hanging out of my swimsuit, but I had no idea because I couldn't feel it. And you know, just things like that that I've gotta just kind of let roll off and laugh about and move on.

Hannah is a young woman in her mid-twenties. For Hannah, the decision to have surgery, complete with her own research about the procedures, was quick. She knew she wanted to "proceed and get it done with and move on."

The recovery, however, was a longer process, and one that was "more tough mentally than physically." Although she initially felt comfortable with her decisions, a couple months after the procedure "it just hit me and I had a very tough time with it." Because she had surgery at such a young age, Hannah struggles with how this affects her relationships with her peers, because "people aren't even thinking about stuff like this" at her age. This has all been part of her road to recovery, as she tries to move on to the next phase in her life.

Getting to a "new normal" means integrating into their identities and lives the physical, social, and emotional changes women experience as a result of being a BRCA-positive mutation carrier. For most women, it means coming to terms with their post–surgical bodies—with having one breast, no breasts, or reconstructed breasts; with their abdominal scars or swollen arms from lymphedema; or with a lack of estrogen, which can affect their minds and moods and sex lives, as well as their health and looks. It can also mean finding a way to rebuild their emotional lives in the wake of broken family ties, sometimes a consequence of revealing a BRCA-positive mutation status to loved ones. For others, finding a new normal means struggling to forgive important family members. Perhaps a sister or husband withdrew and failed to offer emotional support or care, leaving the BRCA-positive mutation woman feeling isolated and despondent throughout her surgical procedure and recovery. For one woman, it might mean first and foremost that her cancer risk is behind her, which is a big part of Hannah's story. Another woman might incorporate her cancer risk and BRCA-positive mutation status into her identity by blogging about her post–treatment life, working to improve the choices open to her newly diagnosed "sisters," or advocating for medical changes so those with this genetic mutation will be better served. What many women struggle with is to negotiate a space in which being positive for the BRCA mutation remains part of them but is not all consuming. And what about the women I interviewed? When I asked them they noted that the average percentage of their lives taken up by the BRCA experience is 32 percent. But these women were at many different points along their journey, and their individual responses ranged from 2 percent to 96 percent.

Getting to a new normal is an ever-evolving and fluid process. And women use this normalization process to empower themselves and to claim some control over their post–surgical lives. Although chasing the new normal is not quite the same experience for all women, we can nevertheless observe some distinct pathways in their journeys. For women who elect preventive surgery, a first step is learning to be comfortable in their new bodies. But each woman has to look at the big picture at some time: she has to decide how to incorporate her BRCA-positive mutation status and all it entails into her identity. This chapter explores these processes.

Getting to a "New Normal" Post–Surgical Body

Post–surgical women follow their unique pathways to a new normal for years, and many are still travelling these paths. The support and affirmation of family and friends can help along the way. To what extent do women feel that others accept their new bodies? For example, do women who are married or in serious relationships receive acceptance and affirmation from their loved ones? Do they feel their bodies look normal to the outside world? Do they feel those that matter in their lives have given them support and care during their surgeries and recoveries? Do they have the economic resources to sustain their new lives, especially when recovery has been slow, putting increasing economic demands on them and their families?

All these issues promote or hinder how satisfied a woman feels about her reconstructed body, especially if her physical appearance is tightly tied to her identity and sense of femininity. Women who feel uncomfortable or unhappy after surgery, either because they didn't have the specific surgical procedure they wanted or because they are disappointed by its results, may find the journey to a new normal difficult and long. Cynthia, for example, who spoke to me ten years after she'd had a double mastectomy, regrets not sparing her nipples.

> When I realized that they had to take the nipples, it really horrified me at first. And I went to several doctors, several breast surgeons, and asked them if they could do it any way by sparing the nipples. And they all pulled out old research studies showing me that if they do this . . . they might as well not do it [surgery] at all because too many women get breast cancer from it. I was just told, "No. You know, I'm not going to even do that for you. If you want it, I'm not going to do it because it's not safe."

Cynthia worries more, though, about her breast implants. She thinks they don't really fit her body size: "I feel like, um, they're not quite, you know, they don't quite fit. Implants don't fit like normal breasts. So when I look at pictures of myself, it does bother me a little bit. It does bother me that . . .

they look fake or odd." Cynthia has already had multiple surgeries on her breasts, to make them look better and more alike. But after six attempts, she is tired of trying to make them "perfect." She's also struggled with unexpected weight gain, which she puts down to her changed metabolism, the consequence of an oophorectomy.

How much a woman identified with her presurgical body is a powerful influence on how difficult accepting a new normal will be. Women who experience their breasts or ovaries as central to their identities may need to grieve for whatever body part they've lost before they can move on. Stephanie had an easier time than many. From an early age, Stephanie knew about the strong history of breast cancer in her family. Even as a young adult, she'd decided that she would probably need to have her breasts removed, so she spent her younger years minimizing their importance to her. When I asked her how she felt about getting a double mastectomy, she replied, "They're just boobs. I don't need 'em." Over time, women like Stephanie come to see their breasts or ovaries as enemies that will eventually kill them. Very often, women spoke about this using military metaphors, such as "my breasts are ticking time bombs," to convey that they are at war with these body parts. Such imagery allows BRCA-positive women to come to terms more easily with the losses surgery brings. As one woman said about her breasts, "I just couldn't get them off fast enough."

For other women, however, breasts, ovaries, and other elements of the female reproductive system are essential to their identities. After surgery, they need to mourn the physical and emotional loss of a part of who they are. Carrie is twenty-six years old and single. She is deeply concerned about feeling normal in her post–surgical body. At the time of our interview, she is about to have a double mastectomy and notes that thinking about this surgery has already changed her perspective about her own breasts. Before she would complain that her breasts were "never big enough." Not any longer: "Now they're . . . going to be removed, I love them. . . . I actually appreciate them a lot more now." Carrie is "really worried" about what her body will be like after surgery. So she's chosen a nipple-sparing procedure, even though it leaves her cancer risk slightly higher than it could be. "At twenty-six years old and single," she explains, "that's something I want to maintain." Without nipple sparing, Carrie is unsure whether she could handle surgery and reconstruction. Keeping her nipples is tied inextricably to the idea of "looking normal" post-surgery: "I think that's . . . one thing that's . . . convincing me to do the procedure is that I will look somewhat normal . . . even though there's a scar on it." Her surgeon's confirmation that her post–surgical body will look good helped Carrie stay on target to get her mastectomy. "You'll look better," he assured her. "No guy will know a difference." Carrie is willing to maintain a certain level of cancer risk in order to keep her nipples and look normal, and because she knows she can always have them removed in the future (and, therefore, further reduce that risk).

For some women, it is not looking normal, but being able to have children that is essential to their sense of self. These women struggle to decide whether they should have their ovaries removed. Especially younger women, who foresee the complications of discussing such issues with current or future boyfriends, find this decision difficult. Natalie has a strong history of breast cancer in her family and is currently undergoing surveillance on her breasts and ovaries. When Natalie met with a genetic counselor and oncologist, they discussed when she wanted to have children. Natalie's oncologist wants her to start Tamoxifen (a drug which can help prevent breast cancer in high-risk women) before Natalie turns thirty-five. But, if she wants to have children, she must do so before starting on the drug. This discussion "has given [Natalie] that want to start a family before then."

Such a strict plan, however, is not on course with her current life. Although she has been in a "not very serious" relationship for a couple months and sees "definitely potential for marriage," she feels it's too soon to tell her boyfriend about her BRCA-positive mutation status. Natalie wants to see how the next month goes and how their relationship progresses before she decides when to tell him. She feels a lot of pressure to make a relationship work, though, but "maybe not this particular relationship." She doesn't want to think about their relationship in terms of "we need to do this now"; more than anything, she doesn't want the pressure of her BRCA timeline to push him away or into something more than he wants—to overwhelm him. Natalie is struggling to decide "the right time to bring it up," which she still feels is "a ways away."

Getting Back My Life and Back into My Body

Women who have preventive surgery often face significant challenges in the journey to their new normal. These involve struggling not only with the physical changes that come with surgery, but also with rebuilding their sense of body esteem and sexual identity. Feminine identity in American culture is tightly tied to a woman's body image—a woman must feel feminine in order to feel good about herself. Women's breasts, in particular, are a large part of femininity and can determine how satisfied women feel about their bodies and how much positive affirmation they receive from others. Breasts are also considered vital to sexual pleasure and sexual experience (for a woman and her partner). Other research confirms that coping with their post–mastectomy bodies is one of BRCA-positive mutation women's primary struggles. A study on the message boards on the Facing Our Risk of Cancer Empowered (FORCE) website discovered a number of themes related to BRCA-positive mutation women facing their post–surgery selves, including the "fear of the loss of femininity, sexual attraction, and loss of sexual pleasure" from losing one's breasts (Kenen et al. 2007, 793). Undergoing a double mastectomy is tantamount to threatening a woman's sense of feminine identity. Such a procedure adds to the pursuit of a new normal the reclamation of femininity, sexuality, and self-esteem.

By reconstructing their breasts, women seek to reclaim their femininity and sexuality. For many women, this repossession means taking control of the type of reconstruction they want. Often, a woman wants to make sure her breasts look as natural as is possible. Some women even want to find the good in this difficult situation. They use surgery to enhance their sense of themselves as feminine and attractive sexual beings. As one woman comments, "My body looks better now than I did. Because I was a little overweight and I think I look really good now. . . . I like having my smooth tummy, and I went up a size in my breasts, so I have a little bit bigger breasts, and I'm okay, I'm looking pretty good." She had chosen a reconstruction procedure that includes a tummy tuck. This surgery, popular with other BRCA-positive women, removes fat from the abdomen for use in reconstructing the breasts. It has the added benefit of using women's natural body fat instead of silicone so that their breasts will look more natural. A woman may also decide to spare her nipples so at least part of her breasts will still be natural. All women who elect a mastectomy must decide whether to reconstruct their breasts and which sort of reconstruction surgery to have. They also must consider whether to spare their nipples, have them tattooed on, or do without them. In making these choices, they create for themselves a new normal. They redefine their physical identities.

Susan's struggle to find her new normal cuts deeply: surgery to remove her breasts and uterus led Susan to question what it means to be a woman. She realized that, for her, being a woman hinged on having the physical feminine attributes that enable reproduction—breasts, ovaries, and uterus. When these were gone, she felt as though her ability to "live as a woman" had "just died." "Can you still be a woman if you don't have breasts or a uterus?" she asks. "So much of your identity as a woman is in your breasts, and this uterus is symbolic." By deciding to have only one of her breasts removed, by retaining one of her natural breasts, Susan held on to some semblance of feeling feminine, to her sense of herself as sexually appealing. If she were to lose both breasts, she felt she would have to "walk away from any potential future relationships" because she would be "rejected." "I couldn't imagine . . . anyone being attracted to me . . . without any of those female parts," she explains. With neither of her natural breasts, Susan would feel she was not actually a woman—that she wasn't a sexual being at all.

Susan's story gets at the next stage of reaching a new normal: incorporating a reconstructed body into one's sexuality. After preventive mastectomy, with or without reconstruction, women often feel alienated from their bodies and their sexuality. After all, most have in their minds an image of themselves at their most attractive, whether that vision reflects something once achieved or only dreamed of. Now, if that "perfect body" involves having natural breasts, it is unreachable. These women must reclaim their own sexuality and sexual attractiveness to reach their new normal. And they often need affirmation from significant others and sexual partners. How can a woman reconstitute her sexuality when others define it as having typical female body parts? How can a woman feel sexual without her breasts or when her breasts have lost sensitivity? What if intercourse is difficult or even painful because of vaginal dryness that should not be relieved by hormonal therapy? Can these women learn how to be sexual in a different way?

Tammy, thirty-nine, struggles with her sexuality in the wake of her mastectomy and hysterectomy. "Life is different" after her surgeries, she tells me. "The repercussions of the hysterectomy are still with me in terms of not having my hormones and being in menopause." She continues, "My sexuality and my libido [have] seemingly just been stripped completely." She even questions her identity as female: "Am I still who I was? You know, am I complete? Am I still a woman?" While reaching a new normal remains a struggle, the support of her husband comforts Tammy, especially in light of her own discomfort over what it truly means to be a woman.

Kelly also recalls the importance of her "post–surgical boyfriend," as she calls him, in reclaiming her sexuality and her sense of being physically attractive. Experiencing this man's desire after her double mastectomy was critical in helping her feel like a woman. She met him shortly after her mastectomy. Because he's a painter who "loves women and loves their bodies and does a lot of nude drawing," she explains, he was used to "bodies being imperfect." She was with him for six months and had "the most amazing sexual experiences." "He must have told me a million times how beautiful my breasts are," she recalls. Although the relationship ended, for Kelly, this affirmation of her new body's attractiveness helped her "erase any question as to whether I can feel like a woman again." This man helped Kelly to understand her new body (her reconstructed breasts in particular) in a sexual context. He also showed her she could still have sexual and romantic relationships with men, and that men still accepted, appreciated, and desired her. Kelly now says that she "would love to" start a new relationship and get married. She accepts and claims her new body and her new sexuality as part of her new normal.

Identifying with My Post–Surgical Body

Surgical reconstruction is often a drawn-out process that can take upwards of eighteen months to complete. And it can take even longer for a woman to accept her post–surgical body and her feelings about it. Doing both, however, is part of each woman's process of reaching a new normal. Women often take time to see their current selves as different from their past selves but still *themselves*. For a woman who elects mastectomy and reconstruction, this integration of past and present identity entails incorporating new breasts as a part of her body. Andrea elected to have saline implants, using an expander method, in which her surgeon placed deflated implants into her breasts. These implants were hooked up to tubes left inserted into the side of each breast (called drains) for the monthly addition of saline. She notes that it was easier to feel "bonded" with her breasts because her surgeon used her own skin to cover the implants.

> I felt comfortable with them. I guess you can say I bonded with them. I did grieve for the loss of losing mine, you know? I remember the first time I was walking down the hall from my hospital room after my surgery and that was when I was able to touch myself again and touched my own skin. It took another year probably for them to really feel like me 'cause they're definitely different.

One of my interviewees, Kristin, also had a preventive mastectomy and reconstruction. As a young woman, she had battled eating disorders, so acceptance of her body had long been an issue for her. While her husband's support was very important, a huge turning point for Kristin was getting involved with the Scar Project. This project is an awareness campaign that photographs women with mastectomy scars. According to the project's website, the campaign "puts a raw, unflinching face on early onset breast cancer, while paying tribute to the courage and spirit of so many brave young women" (David Jay Photography 2011). Being photographed with her scars allowed Kristen to gain confidence in herself, and forced her to be "open" about being a BRCA-positive mutation carrier. It was when her photos were going to go public that Kristin realized she could accept her new self.

> I was tired of chasing down this ideal that I knew I could never be anymore. And I just decided, "This is me." [laughing] This—it is what it is, and this is me, and I'm just going to be open with it. And you know, I think there's been events between the surgery and now that have helped me in that direction, but I really think that that was the moment that I decided, "I have got to just accept this as me and be okay with it."

Kristin's journey toward being "okay" with her new body was supported fully by her husband and by the Scar Project. Both allowed her to feel beautiful. And her current state of mind continues to evolve.

> I can deal with it in pieces. And I honestly feel like this has been the year where I've been most accepting of myself. Um, I tend to be a perfectionist, and I think that, for a while, I just could not face that this is it [laughing]. And it's almost like I've relieved myself and I've given myself a new freedom to accept that I will never be perfect in the world's standards, and, well good, because now I don't have to chase that anymore, I can actually enjoy living my life.

Although getting to this new normal was difficult, ultimately, Kristin is happier now than when she was trying to "be perfect in the world's standards." Having said this, I don't see too much about self-love or about Kristin loving her new body in her story; her feelings are more "well, okay then—this is it."

For women who have their ovaries removed, getting to a new normal also means living with the onset of premature menopause. The early onset of menopause means not only becoming infertile, which can be especially difficult for young women, but also a rapid decline in physical well-being. Julia, a thirty-six-year-old, divorced, childless, and "lonely" woman who had a difficult time adjusting to being BRCA positive, struggled with these problems. She "cried every day" for a month and a half after learning her results. She had an oophorectomy, but the decision was traumatic because she didn't want to go through early menopause, and she had still hoped to have children of her own. "I never had any intention of it. But then, just, my one aunt kind of scared me into it by, um, telling me . . . it is so hard to detect [ovarian cancer through surveillance]," Julia says. She said that "a huge weight was lifted off my shoulders" after the surgery, but she remains "so upset about not being able to have children," and "frustrated" because finances prevent her from other reproductive options. Julia exemplifies how difficult it can be to for a woman to come to terms with the removal of her ability to give birth.

Sometimes, identifying with your body is a transcendental experience. A rare experience among the women I interviewed was to reflect on surgical decisions and their new bodies from a religious perspective. Yet some do. They rely not only on the people in their lives but also on God in developing their attitudes about post–testing decisions and physical changes. As one religious Mormon woman told me, "We believe in forever. So we don't believe there's ever a time where that will halt . . . your progression. . . . So having my ovaries removed or having—having a hysterectomy would be a temporal decision for me." When another Mormon woman, Emma, told me her story, I realized how complicated making these temporal decisions can be. Emma is not only deeply reflective about her religious beliefs with regard to how she feels about her body, but she also relies heavily on what others think about her reconstructed body.

Emma's process of reaching some semblance of a new normal and a positive body image currently hinges on the opinions of others, mainly those of her husband and of important figures in her community. She lives in a tightly knit Mormon community where everyone knows about her BRCA-positive status and her decision to have preventive surgeries. "Every single person in my neighborhood knows it's happened," Emma laughs. "I've had advice from various people on what size to go." Her husband wants her looking as "normal" as possible. Her neighbors have variously commented on the potential size of her reconstructed breasts. Her plastic surgeon told her, "You know what, it's really important to me that you look normal." Her reconstruction has almost becomes a social project in which her decisions are shaped by several layers of social input. If it were up to Emma, she would not have any reconstruction. "I'll do it because it's not that big a deal for me," she explains. "But I just thought, well, you know why bother? Um . . . because of loss of sensation and everything else, but I don't really need it."

Emma's decision to go with reconstructed breasts, then, is shaped by the desires of other people that she look like a "normal" female. Her reconstruction process becomes a social project driven not by her own desire, for, as she says, her new normal is what others think it should be. Personally, Emma feels there will be nothing left inside of her (breasts and ovaries) to make her a woman after her surgery. She notes in the next breath, however, that she is not overly concerned with her body image in its connection to her feminine identity. Emma remains positive because of her Mormon faith, which includes the belief that everyone comes back in the next life in a "perfect state." So, whatever happens to her in this life, ultimately, she will have and looks forward to identifying with her perfect body in the afterlife.

On the other hand, some women feel no pressure to incorporate what other people think their new normal should be. Instead, they aim to feel comfortable and normal with the scars and the loss of their breasts or the loss of their natural breasts. One woman who opted for breast reconstruction without nipple sparing or nipple reconstruction describes looking down at her breasts and connecting them with "a positive mental connotation." She doesn't miss her nipples, and her scars remind her of her victory—she's taken steps to prevent breast cancer. One study found that women had diverse experiences reaching towards accepting their new bodies and selves, yet all had to "renegotiate their identity where they felt less of a woman, and accommodate a new identity with significantly reduced cancer risk" (Lloyd et al. 2000, 482). Each woman takes unique path to reach her new normal, where she can be comfortable in her own skin.

Finding a New Normal in Relationships and Identity

Finding a new normal transcends the physical and reaches into a woman's personal relationships with others and with herself. It is constituted by her emotional life, the quality of her connections to family and friends, and how relationships change for good and bad in her transition from pre- to post–BRCA testing and diagnosis life. When women feel supported by those close to them, their transition can be easier and more fulfilling. However, sometimes, getting to a new normal means addressing the emotional self—for example, a difficult marriage or loneliness. For a few women in my study, such as Andrea's story later on in this chapter, this reexamination of their lives and emotional health has led to the severing of close relationships.

For all the women in my study, being diagnosed with the BRCA mutation means finding a place in their lives for that genetic status and for the risks and decisions it entails. Some women take preventive steps and move past the BRCA-positive mutation diagnosis. Thinking they have defeated their cancer risk, these women see BRCA as only a small part of who they are. Others remain in turmoil from the news; they think about their BRCA status daily and incorporate it into their lives and identities. In studying women's conversations on the FORCE website, it was found that BRCA-positive women tend to wind up in a state of "chronic risk" (Kenen et al. 2007, 796). They "are trying to prevent their past and future from consuming them" and to accept preventive surgery in order to guarantee their future (Kenen et al. 2007, 796). Most women seek to strike some balance; they recognize that they are BRCA positive but don't let the fact consume them. Many women take on the identity of "previvor," a term I discuss later.

Even women who choose surveillance rather than preventative surgery must work to integrate their cancer risk status into otherwise normal lives. They do not want their genetic status to define their identities, so they are willing to grant BRCA only a small but continuous presence in their lives. Regular screening becomes part of their new normal. Past research also supports the conclusion that most women, even if they struggle along the way, find contentment in their identity as a BRCA-positive woman and in the decisions they make. One study on emotions and stigma among BRCA-positive women found that, overall, these women had high self-esteem (Vodermaier, Esplen, and Maheu 2010). In fact, their anxiety over cancer was not determined by how long ago they had been diagnosed as having the BRCA gene, but was related to other factors, for example, their family history of cancer. Additionally, women were very satisfied with preventive surgery, and those who decide to have BRCA testing are a "self-selected sample and may have accepted the possibility of prophylactic surgery" (Vodermaier, Esplen, and Maheu 2010, 308). While women wait until they are ready to get tested and have surgery, once they *are* ready, they are confident in their decisions and able to maintain high self-esteem and confidence in them.

Women, too, see the process of reaching a new normal as ongoing. They seek to address their cancer risk actively and move beyond it: "I accept the strong pull of my BRCA diagnosis and will deal with it. I want to start the next phase of my life." The term *new normal* comes from the BRCA-positive mutation women themselves. It's how they define their transitional journey. As one of the women I interviewed puts it, "I'm just trying to come to terms with what my new normal was going to be . . . because I knew I was going to do the surgeries, but it's like, 'Well, what is that new normal, and how do I come to accept it?'" Another explains, "But I'm getting through a lot of [the challenges of being BRCA-positive mutation carrier and having surgery], especially now that I'm, you know, done with the reconstruction, and I'm at, . . . quote unquote, 'my new normal.' But it gets better, it definitely gets better."

Reassessing Marriage: Andrea's Story

For Andrea, and a few other women in my study, reaching a new normal meant standing up for themselves and ending unhealthy relationships. Andrea experienced her BRCA diagnosis as the final straw. Her husband's unsupportive and uncaring attitude had brought her to the breaking point when she was first diagnosed with cancer and had to undergo chemotherapy. Later, while suffering the trauma of a preventive double mastectomy and hysterectomy, she broke. At the age of forty, with her cancer treatment and surgery behind her and a twelve-year-old daughter to care for, she ended her unhappy marriage of twenty-one years.

Andrea describes her husband as especially selfish during the time she was diagnosed with cancer, underwent chemotherapy, and discovered her BRCA-positive status.

> He wasn't going to go out of his way, um, too much. I mean, he's a nice man and all that stuff, but he's probably stuck at around fifteen, sixteen years old emotionally. . . . Like when I was bald, that was a big issue for me. That was, that was probably one of the hardest parts was losing my hair. And I would always ask him and my daughter, please just knock on my door before you come in. You know, I'll put a scarf on. I'll put something on. This was for me. And he would just never do that. He would just come right in. We got in this argument about it. He says, "I'm try- you know, it's not important to me, it doesn't matter to me." And I appreciate that, but it really matters to me. He wasn't listening to me.

When I ask Andrea what her husband could have done to be more supportive for her, she answers with two main points—respecting her wishes and helping take care of their daughter. During her recovery, Andrea, who was used to cooking dinner and cleaning the house, felt upset about not being healthy enough to fulfill her role in the home and as a parent: "I was sad not to be able to do the things I would do with her, for her." Her husband didn't pick up the slack. He didn't take over her duties, which hindered her own healing process. Andrea thinks he did not come through for her in the way she had expected. Sometimes, he seemed downright callous and oblivious of her feelings as a BRCA-positive mutation cancer survivor.

> His life went on fine and he, you know, into the Harleys, into the motorcycles, whatever. And he had been to the Halloween party or something, and he was getting dressed up and going in drag or some weird thing with his leather chaps. And he's like, "Hey!" He tells me, "Let me borrow your wig." And he puts on my wig, and he just thinks it's hysterical. I start crying, and he's like, and I was mad. I wasn't crying; I was just mad. I was being bitchy. And he's like, "You know Andrea, what's the deal? You know, just go and have a good time." And I was like, you know, you just don't get it. See this wig, I say. I have to wear this wig every day so I don't feel like a freak, and you're putting it on like a joke.

Being diagnosed with cancer and the BRCA mutation, undergoing chemotherapy, and the invasive preventive surgeries to address her risk of cancer were challenging milestones in Andrea's life. Her husband did not recognize even that Andrea had deep feelings about her experiences. In a marriage, which should be mutually supporting, this ignorance is destructive and hurtful.

Perhaps the couple could have worked through his thoughtlessness had they built up a store of kind and loving memories, but the relationship was in trouble before any BRCA-related issues surfaced: "This was gonna be the test you know? Twenty-one years of life together." Her husband's failure to come through was the breaking point in their marriage. Now that they have separated, she is glad that her experiences empowered to get out of an unhealthy marriage.

> I was ready to move on. You know when something like cancer and my surgery happens, your perspective just so changes, you know? I mean, what if I was gonna die in five years? This is not, I'm not gonna waste five years more. I'm forty years old, and then my dad got diagnosed. My dad dies, like, next year, then the divorce. It was a lot going on. Sold the house, moved, did a lot within these four years. I am in a better place. I'd rather be alone than be with a guy that's just a jerk. My illness was a gift. It was a wake up.

Becoming a Previvor

For some of the women in my study, part of coming to terms with their BRCA-positive status is taking on the bodily or somatic identity of "previvor." This label, derived from the prefix *pre* (meaning *before*) and the last part of the word, *survivor,* was developed by communities of BRCA-positive women to describe themselves—people who tackle and survive cancer before it strikes. The term was first used on the message boards of FORCE's website. BRCA-positive women felt the need for a word to describe the experiences of living with the risk of hereditary breast and ovarian cancer, and the term *previvor* was coined ("Cancer Previvors: Overview").

In sociology, the term *biosociality* is often used to describe the behavioral changes that individuals with a specific medical and/or genetic risk conditions begin to express, by embodying and relating to their genetic risk status and/or genetic code. Some may go on to form social communities, where individual members take on unique biosocial identities that are associated with these genetic conditions. These newly formed biosocialities are in turn supported, and reaffirmed, by medical specialists and genetics, as well as by their online genetic community counselors (Rabinow 1992; Atkinson, Greenslade, and Glasner 2007; Gibbon and Novas 2008; Gibbon 2008).

Taking on the previvor identity can be very powerful and affirming. Liz, whose story in chapter 5 detailed her decision to have preventative surgery, was inspired to create a website devoted to the concerns of previvors. For her, she described how being a previvor asserts control—she has "taken something negative and turn[ed] it into positive." Her website empowers other women in similar situations by allowing them to talk through their problems in an uplifting and proactive way. Because Liz did not have support from other BRCA-positive women, she "had no one to talk to" about being BRCA positive or preventive options. Her own lack of support drove her, through the website, to be a resource for women in similar situations. It also allows Liz to stay invested in her own identity as a BRCA-positive woman, and to ensure this identity will remain a part of her life.

Giving back to the previvor community becomes, for many women, an important way of reaching their new normal. Many are active in online or face-to-face communities, exchanging messages, attending in-person and virtual meetings and conferences. Tammy participates in FORCE initiatives; the organization hosts an online forum as well as local events and larger conferences to provide a wide range of support for BRCA-positive mutation women. Tammy did "research on the FORCE website [and] . . .

attended the FORCE conference," which was the turning point for her to realize she wanted a preventive mastectomy. Tammy started working to create a FORCE chapter in her city, and, after having preventive surgery, she "started to get very involved with FORCE. . . . And it was kind of—it was very therapeutic because it just helped kind of bring everything full circle." Tammy uses FORCE not only as a site for information and support but also as a way of giving back to the BRCA community.

Others are so affected by their experience that it begins to change their career paths. Some women become genetic counselors or get involved in the medical profession in some way. Melissa began marketing the "spa bra" in her business after her very painful recovery from breast surgery. She sees selling this product as a way to alleviate some of the pain for other women who choose mastectomy, as well as a fundraising opportunity for the cause.

> With how uncomfortable it was, um, with the expanders, that actually one of our products was phenomenal. And it's called the spa bra. And I could wear it from the very beginning. And I was shocked. Because when you have a [prophylactic bilateral mastectomy] your nerves are just on fire, and it's so uncomfortable, and you don't want anything on your skin, but you need something. So I thought . . . I could possibly market it to a mastectomy shop. And then I realized as I was going through these procedures and going through the different websites, that, wow, there's a lot of fundraising that actually takes place. . . . and I thought, why not combine the spa bra with fundraising? It's the same model with direct sales, except people, you know, volunteers, can sell the spa bra . . . and they can earn 50 for their charity.

Many BRCA-positive mutation women work hard to make something positive out of their own difficult experiences, whether that means fundraising, selling specialty products, or choosing a career or volunteer work that will benefit other previvors. "I decided to channel all of that, um, kind of that angst, and kind of feeling helpless," Melissa notes. "And I'm like, well, let's do something positive with it."

While connecting with the wider BRCA community, these women take on the previvor identity in order to validate the experience of facing their risk of cancer and taking action. They give this experience a name and acknowledge it, recognizing that, even though they aren't necessarily cancer survivors, they have persevered through huge challenges in confronting their BRCA-positive mutation status.

Previvorhood as a Lifestyle: Erica's Story

Erica embraces previvorhood. She accepts her BRCA status, telling me, "It will always be a part of my identity." Currently in her late thirties, Erica recently underwent a double mastectomy. As she explains it, her identity as a previvor was solidified as she sought support from online communities.

> I spent a lot of time especially leading up to surgery on the Internet. I asked a lot of questions, got incredible info. I really like the website's young previvor forum. I resonated with the term previvor because women live with this condition of having BRCA-positive gene mutation. Some of their stories were scary, but comforting, and honest. On the website, women are communicating and reaching out to each other, saying, "You're gonna be okay." It was very supportive.

Erica strongly identifies with being a previvor, having had preventative breast and ovarian surgeries in her early thirties. As Erica sees things, neither her husband nor her parents have offered much emotional support. In fact, her parents haven't spoken to her at all since she's had surgery. So Erica comforts herself by reaching out to cancer support groups, and she belongs to several online cancer communities that accept her condition and her decisions. Going online and reading about women whose cancer stories are "more positive" is a good experience for Erica, as these women have also been on this precancer journey.

Assuming the identity of a previvor is "crucial" to Erica's "survival." Erica thinks it's "dangerous" for BRCA-positive mutation women to have their surgeries and then think no more about their risk. After all, they still have the gene. In her opinion, a BRCA-positive diagnosis means living with "stage zero cancer" for life. So these individuals need to "make the right choices" throughout their lives to prevent cancer, such as eating healthily, watching their caffeine intake, and exercising.

Erica identifies problems within the previvor community, however. She thinks many previvors just take without giving back, by lurking on the edges of forums or harvesting information from websites. Or they feel superior to cancer survivors because previvors were proactive about their health and so didn't get cancer. She is particularly upset when individuals criticize previvors for focusing too much on their cancer risk. For example, a young woman she met at a conference provoked Erica's anger by proclaiming to the other previvors, "I don't have cancer. You all need to move on. You don't either." She thinks this attitude stems from denial: "They just want to believe what they want to believe, and they don't look at the reality" of being BRCA positive for life. Previvors also experience pushback from the outside, according to Erica. For example, she feels that previvors' concerns are often dismissed in the cancer community as a whole. In fact, she sees a split in this community between being a "previvor and survivor," and she's noticed a "strong attitude among survivors that trivializes being a previvor," who hasn't "been through the same war"—the chemotherapy and radiation treatments—as a survivor. Despite ambivalence about the purpose and meaning of the term *previvor* and its implications for how BRCA-positive women frame their experiences, Erica and other women are uplifted by this identity because it allows them to acknowledge the difficulty of their experiences and join a community to work together to address their cancer risk.

Struggling to Find a New Normal: Amelia's Story

Some of the women I interviewed had a difficult time reaching their new normal. Some had not reached it. As women struggle to reconcile themselves with their new circumstances, many face challenges within themselves and within their relationships—challenges that seem insurmountable. Amelia has not yet come to terms with being BRCA positive. She is thirty-five and recently divorced, and she has had an oophorectomy and hysterectomy. She easily made the decision to remove her ovaries, possibly because she already has a five-year-old son. But she's ignored the recommendation to have a mastectomy. Amelia shows how tightly her fear and anxiety about having her breasts removed is linked to the crisis of femininity she expects after undergoing preventative surgery: "We're removing our femininity, we're removing parts of our body. . . . Society . . . sexualizes the breasts so much. . . . It's very heavy stuff." Amelia has trouble even thinking about this surgery. Her oophorectomy and hysterectomy have brought on early menopause, so she's already struggling with body issues.

> I've been dealing with symptoms of menopause now [laughs] at thirty-eight, and, you know, I'm, I'm finding myself, you know, gaining weight and . . . my hair has changed, my skin's changing, I'm getting a, a mustache [laughs] you know? . . . And losing your breasts on top of that is like a cruel. . . . It's like, how much . . . you know, can my self-esteem handle? How much can—? And right now, you know, I've

taken a break. . . . I dated a little bit. And I've just taken a break. I've just taken myself away from that, you know. I'm not ready.

Amelia continues to struggle with being BRCA-positive mutation carrier. From day to day, its significance changes for her: "some days, you know, some days it might be 1 percent. Some days it might be 99.9 [laughs]." But, as she explains, knowledge of her genetic mutation and its repercussions for herself and her son is a constant part of her life: "something I, I live with and think about every day. I just, I refuse to say that it defines me, but it certainly has changed me forever."

Yet Amelia hopes this change will not necessarily be a detrimental one. She discusses her mastectomy not only as a preventative measure but also as something that can improve her body image and self-esteem.

> I've really been interested in looking into this [new breast reconstruction procedure]. . . . They take from your, your stomach. . . . They basically take fat . . . and reconstruct and . . . now that I've had a C-section and a hysterectomy, my stomach is definitely not what it used to be. And that would be . . . [a] tummy tuck and a . . . boob job at the same time. This might not be so bad [laughs]. . . . Maybe I'll get my self-esteem back.

Finding a New Normal after BRCA and Cancer: Diane's Story

Although all the women I interviewed have to at least acknowledge their BRCA-positive mutation status, this process can become even more complicated for women who have also been diagnosed with cancer, especially for those who have been diagnosed with stage IV cancer. A research analysis on the experiences of women with breast cancer showed that as women slowly progress through stages of suffering and transformation, they sometimes are "feeling stuck" in facing their diagnosis. However, women can and do "transform the cancer experience from threat to possible meaning" (Arman and Rehnsfeldt 2003, 521). Diane's story shows this, how cancer survivors in particular can redefine themselves and their experiences in a positive way.

Diane was in shock for weeks after learning she was positive for the BRCA mutation, and she struggled to maintain her self-esteem throughout her mastectomy and chemotherapy, which were "devastating to my psyche."

She also faced financial issues due to poor insurance coverage, and at the time of my interview she told me she still owed about $30,000 for her medical bills. But Diane feels very empowered by her experiences, and she is proud of what she has overcome. She is "very healthy" and living a new normal life again, and she has made her BRCA-mutation diagnosis and cancer experiences into "more of a positive thing for me," by joining the Pink Ribbon Cowgirls, a group of breast cancer survivors in Texas who host meetings, fundraising events, and social gatherings. Diane told me she is not defined by BRCA or cancer, but that she finds her identity by making something good come of both: "It's exhilarating. I just, I feel empowered, like I feel powerful. I feel like I have conquered the world." Women like Diane turn the extreme circumstances of both being BRCA positive and a cancer survivor into a positive experience, both for themselves and for others in their lives. Diane told me, "I wasn't going to let it stop me live my life . . . I really don't want to make my life about the fact that I had cancer."

Life After Stage IV Cancer: Cassandra's Story

One woman's story affected me more than most. At the time of our interview, Cassandra had experienced two occurrences of breast cancer, first in 2001 and a reoccurrence of stage IV cancer in 2004. I wasn't expecting to be so profoundly moved by this interview, but I vividly remember it. Cassandra was one of the few women I spoke with who was at stage IV breast cancer. And my younger sister had been given the same diagnosis. When Cassandra and I spoke, there was not one part of my sister's body that was not invaded by cancer. So I already had very definite, but very stereotyped, views about what that diagnosis meant: I thought both women were waiting to die. So how could I ask Cassandra about her new identity after surgery and chemotherapy? For me, that question made no sense, given my own experiences with my sister. As far as I understood, stage IV meant preparing to die, not recalibrating your life. Cassandra told me that when others ask about how she is doing in front of her young children, she starts to cry, and she feels as if she is about "to fall off the cliff." But, while listening to Cassandra's story, I realized that her life is not yet about dying: it's about living with a new normal, even in the face of a terminal illness.

Cassandra says her journey is not about waging war; rather, it contains many elements of hide-and-seek. Her cancer is hiding and mutating, and it is her job to snuff it out, to find it and destroy it before it destroys her. So she fills her days with creative ways of continuing to live: brainstorming about new chemotherapy medications that might work when the old ones give out, working with her oncologist to watch for cancer reoccurrences, staving off death by knowing when to get a CT scan to avoid radiation overdoses, and saving radiation treatments for when they count.

Luckily, Cassandra has an incredible support system, an army of women who, like Cassandra, have stage IV cancer and are making a last stand together. For Cassandra, her new normal life is an ongoing process.

> When you're in an earlier stage [of cancer] . . . what you think is, "I just want to get the hell out of Dodge." You know, you want to get your treatment and you want to get the hell out of Dodge. But when you're Stage IV you never get out of Dodge. And not only do you not get out of Dodge, but you find that you just bought a condominium in Dodge. A condominium with no resale value. And you can't get out of Dodge. And you look around at some point, in this condominium in this city [where] you really don't want to live. It—you see that you have these neighbors. And you say, "Even though this place totally sucks, I am so glad you're my neighbor."

Cassandra calls her fellow stage IV women "IV Leaguers," which is "a triple entendre because it's like the IV, and of course the Ivy League, but also stage four is I-V." These are the women who also live in Dodge and with whom she can make her last stand. Together, they want to be at peace, but they also to show the world that there *is* life after a stage IV diagnosis. The IV Leaguers are her neighbors. "We throw parties. We celebrate our still living here. We know no one can really leave here except if they die." They throw these events to promote awareness: "so people can see us and people like me, who are diagnosed, [who] don't immediately equate it with death. Instead they equate it with a possibility that they're going to live, and that there are people that—who they can contact that can help them."

Creating this community and accepting their diagnoses makes living with stage IV some kind of "normal." As Cassandra explains, this support system is crucial in the fight.

> In Dodge City, of course we can leave and go see our supporters— those in the medical community who help us to remain in Dodge. For example, our oncologist becomes our copilot, our friend, and maybe even someone we have a huge crush on. The pharmacist who keeps our

medicine chest filled. . . . We have an extended community of medical helpers who keep us abreast of what new goodies we can place in our medicine chest. We also have each other—the members who reside in our Dodge City condominium apartment complex.

The knowledge that so many women are in this together with her comforts Cassandra, who also realizes the stark, unfortunate reality of her circumstances, with no end date for her "perpetual treatment." When I asked Cassandra how a woman rebuilds her life after a stage IV diagnosis, she told me that ultimately, it is all about having "a balance between ignorance and knowledge as well as acceptance and denial." She thinks this balancing act is essential not only for women at her stage of cancer, but also for all BRCA-positive women at every stage of their journey. In order to balance, Cassandra must accept that she needs treatment in order to continue her life. "When treatment has ended," she explains, "we know our days in Dodge are marked." Dodge City, then, is both a consolation, and a reminder of the new normal in which she now resides.

Conclusion: Still Waiting for Cancer to Come?

This chapter outlines a remarkable journey, one that BRCA-positive mutation women take as they seek a new normal in their lives. Each woman's path is different, but they all must come to terms with their emotional selves, and they must adjust their relationships with friends and family members, networks that are often reconfigured during a woman's BRCA experience. Some women struggle to reconnect with their post–surgical bodies and to integrate their physical changes into their new sense of femininity and sexuality. Some women must overcome enormous obstacles before reaching their new normal. Some women never reach it. For women like Cassandra and her IV Leaguers, the new normal changes each day, as they seek out innovative cancer treatments that let them live—in both denial and awareness of impending death. For many previvors, reaching the new normal means laying all fear of cancer to rest—no longer are they waiting for cancer to come. For other women, they reach their new normal by accepting and living with that fear—or even with the certainty that cancer will kill them.

Although not all BRCA-positive mutation women feel as strongly as others that they are just waiting for cancer to come, it is a fear each woman faces. Acknowledging this fear is a step along the path to a new identity, to a new normal not only for a woman with this genetic risk but also for her family. It is important to recognize that BRCA has implications for present *and* future generations. One study found that children who grow up knowing of their family's breast cancer risk and BRCA-positive mutation history do worry about their own and their family's health and, overwhelmingly, want to undergo genetic testing themselves in the future (Tercyak et al. 2001). So finding a new normal may mean addressing the fears of family members as well: perhaps a BRCA-positive woman's children or grandchildren; perhaps siblings, aunts, and uncles, some of whom do not want to get tested; perhaps others who are still too young or who refuse to acknowledge the cancer risk.

The repercussions of BRCA testing and from BRCA-positive mutation diagnoses reach even farther, however. Enhanced individualized risk assessment and the fears and treatment expectations arising from genetic testing have societal effects and bring to mind broad questions. For example, what large-scale social changes and social-policy actions can make being positive for the BRCA mutation more empowering for women? What should we, as a society, do after listening to these women's stories? What issues and concerns do BRCA-positive women express concerning their social interactions and medical treatment? And what voices have been left out of this and other BRCA narratives, such as men who are at risk, or women who cannot afford to get tested? Finally, what role should the genetic testing industry play? What changes may be needed to make genetic testing more affordable to those who are at risk, and how can this be done without alarming women who do need to become part of the testing culture? These wider issues are the focus of the next chapter.

SEVEN

Toward Empowerment

"I accept the strong pull of my BRCA diagnosis and will deal with it. I want to start the next phase of my life."

BRCA-positive mutation women seek to empower themselves, to get on with enjoying full and fulfilling lives in spite of the news that they carry the BRCA mutation. The stories that I was fortunate enough to hear and share with you reveal women talking back to their BRCA diagnosis, maintaining hope for the future, and finding ways to move forward with their lives.

Gaining Personal Empowerment

One important way women empower themselves is by establishing a new normal—a fresh identity, an orientation that allows each woman to continue accomplishing her goals while finding a place (large or small) for the BRCA-positive mutation in her life. What this "normal life" becomes varies based on the quality of support within each woman's network of social relationships, as well as her particular stage of life in terms of age, marital status, and children. There are other crucial factors: a woman's perception of her risk of getting or dying from cancer; whether there is a strong history of cancer in her family; whether she already has cancer, and how aggressive and advanced it is. Experiences also vary according to whether BRCA-positive women have easy access to the medical assistance and economic resources they need to reach their new normal.

In interviews, women made it clear to me that the quality of their BRCA experience depends on more than whether they get cancer. This observation is logical when we understand that these women are at different life stages, and they have different perspectives on their cancer risk. For some, any risk is too great and any wait to minimize that risk is too long. These women opt for preventive surgery as soon as possible. They live in fear that their breasts are ticking time bombs waiting to go off, and surgery is a tool of empowerment that will help them gain a new lease on life.

For other women, electing to have surgery to minimize their cancer risk is not that simple. They are not ready to have surgery and do not necessarily see a surgical option as empowering, given their present life circumstances. In fact, as we have observed, some women avoid confirming their BRCA-mutation status by delaying the initial test. Their unpreparedness serves as a protective strategy; they only learn their test results when they can face them and take steps toward empowerment. Take the case of one woman who originally heard about her family history and the BRCA test when she was in graduate school and trying to get pregnant. "I thought I would wait to actually find out until I was done with my childbearing years," she says. In a similar vein, Christina recalls her decision to wait to get tested.

> The test is so decisive. . . . At the end of it . . . if you have this—these horrible chances of getting cancer, or if you don't. . . . I think that waiting helped me get used to the idea that . . . this mastectomy could be the ultimate outcome. . . . It felt too young for me to have to be thinking about stuff like this. . . . I wasn't ready. I wasn't married. I was living in a group apartment with my fiancé, and . . . one of my best friends. . . . I was sort of doing the grad school thing, so there was the sense that . . . it was too early to have all of this medical information . . . interloping on my life. I knew that, and I also knew that knowing would sort of change me and change my life. . . . I was really happy where I was . . . at that moment. And I didn't want to do anything to spoil that.

These women recognize that they are not ready to take the preventive steps necessary to address their cancer risk if they are BRCA-positive mutation carriers, so they empower themselves by making the decision to postpone testing until they are ready to take action.

Some women, after testing positive for the BRCA mutation, begin a self-imposed waiting game. They carefully monitor their bodies using a variety of surveillance tests and calibrate the amount of time they *think* they have before cancer *might* strike, basing these estimations on the cancer history of their families. When did mom die? How old was my sister when she was diagnosed? These women elect to elevate life goals like careers and families that would be directly affected by preventive surgery. They are willing to negotiate for time before they think about their cancer risk. They also buy time by meticulously planning future surgical procedures. In one instance, a woman took charge of her surgical experience by carefully planning what "chunk" of her life "away from dating and meeting people" would be dedicated to surgery. She didn't feel she was "going to be . . . mentally, emotionally able to . . . date until" all surgical procedures were completed. More broadly, for women who are at high risk for ovarian cancer, this planning may mean having their ovaries removed first and choosing surveillance for their breasts. Again, family history is a crucial factor that helps each woman determine the timing of her surgical procedures. The waiting game can become easily upended if a woman is diagnosed with cancer—this diagnosis will, at least temporarily, overshadow other goals as surviving cancer now takes top priority.

How a woman experiences her BRCA-positive mutation diagnosis depends on more than just her nature and character. Her path is more than a personal response or choice and is affected directly by family members. How relatives receive or respond to a woman's diagnosis, particularly the amount of isolating behaviors or support they provide, is a critical element in whether or not women have an empowering experience. Erica suffered a "bit of depression" over the lack of emotional support from her husband and family. On the other hand, families who reach out and provide support and guidance often enhance a woman's sense of empowerment. She feels buttressed and more able to handle the challenges arising at different stages in her BRCA journey. A supportive network of other BRCA-positive mutation women, who have already gone through many of these challenges, can also make the journey less isolating. But a close family member or loved one—a supportive husband, sister, or boyfriend who is present not only physically but also emotionally—can be essential to empowerment. That is because feeling empowered also means taking up the challenge of creating a new normal, and the emotional support of at least one significant other can be critical to achieving the affirmation and acceptance of this new normal, this new identity.

Previous research shows that family history is a critical filter women use to assess the risk information they receive from medical personnel (Hallowell and Lawton 2002; Kenen et al. 2003). Yet it is not only their personal networks of support that are critical in moving women towards a sense of empowerment. The quality of medical advice, care, and resources that they receive from health-care providers and organizations affects their sense of empowerment as well. Thus, it is essential for care providers to understand decision-making from women's perspectives and to discover those factors within the medical environment that serve to empower or disempower this decision making.

How Can Medical Systems Empower Women?

The women I interviewed had plenty of ideas about what they would like to change in the health-care system—about how to make it work better for those who are BRCA-positive mutation carriers. These suggestions come directly from their individual experiences. Some women faced financial barriers to good care because of the high cost of BRCA testing and preventative medical procedures. These obstacles often gained muscle because women didn't have health insurance. Many women also worried about the lack of a patient-centered approach among health-care providers, whom they accused of not understanding their lived experience of carrying the BRCA mutation. The medical-centered perspective most of my interviewees encountered tended to place them in a diagnostic one-size-fits-all box, leaving them feeling disempowered in their interactions with medical personnel. These women's stories illuminate the ways in which the medical professionals and health-care system can be altered in order to improve the unique concerns and circumstances of BRCA-positive women.

Placed in a "Diagnostic Box": Jennifer's Story

Jennifer, whom you remember from chapter 2, used these actual words to describe her disempowering surgical experience, which she told me was "just really not a good experience." She told me her doctors were putting her in a "diagnostic box" instead of looking at her as an individual. They just didn't understand how much pain she was in after her preventive surgery, she felt, and "discouraged [her] from asking questions." She has had a number of surgical complications and poor pain management, all of which caused her considerable discomfort. She notes that she "had to beg and plead for, to stay one night [in the hospital], one more night, and for stronger medication. They wouldn't give me stronger medication." When they finally did, she discovered that she was allergic to the pain medication. Jennifer also thinks she was misled by a physician prior to her surgery. The doctor recommended that she participate in a clinical trial, so she almost took a dangerously high level of what later turned out to be a very toxic drug. She was led to believe that this drug was part of standard treatment protocols when it actually was still being studied.

When she was dissatisfied with her treatment, she reached out and found doctors who listened to her and took a more patient-oriented approach. Jennifer's new doctor expressed anger at her past treatment and contacted her previous clinic. Upon discovering that Jennifer had made a change, her former doctor was upset that she had even looked for a second opinion. Since making the switch, Jennifer feels more comfortable with her treatment, and she has able to have an open dialogue with her providers. Her story clearly points to the need for doctors to listen carefully to patients, be open about procedures and risks, and encourage patients to take control of their own medical decisions.

"A Lot That They Could Improve On": Sam's Story

Some women complained that medical personnel, from genetic counselors to oncologists, lacked knowledge about management and treatment protocols for BRCA mutation carriers. For example, Sam thinks that, in general, "genetic counselors . . . have a lot they could improve on in the way that they tell people" about their positive BRCA-mutation status. Sam was given only the "bare minimum" when she received her positive test results: "I got an envelope with one piece of paper inside that said. . . . 'You have a genetic mutation that could this, this, and this. . . .' There's no information that goes along with it . . . you just get this letter and that's it." Sam had to rely on her own resourcefulness in order to figure out what her positive test result meant for her health. Of the letter she received informing her of her results, Sam told me how she struggled to understand it.

> It's not in English. No one understands what that thing says. I had no idea what it said. I remember when I first got it, I sat there and I was like Googling each word to try to figure out what exactly it meant. . . . Then they're like, "Let me draw you a picture." And you're like, "A picture cannot save this right now. It's already done, I'm confused already."

Processing the result, therefore, can include a degree of translation. And it is a bit much to expect a patient who has just had a shock regarding her health to have to research each unfamiliar medical-scientific term. When Sam received her results, her genetic counselor did not adequately explain them, and she had to interpret the information by herself using the Internet; now, she says, there are "more resources"—although, these resources may not necessarily be located in medical institutions, such as her response that it wasn't until she watched the documentary *In the Family* that she was realized, "Oh, now I get it!" Sam described her surgeon as "great," and "amazing," and explained how "lucky" she was to have her. Yet, despite her overall good experience, she told me, "I think [the genetic counselors] get a bad rap sometimes, but I do think that they have a lot that they could improve on in the way that they tell people."

"I'm Really Scared": Alana's Story

Alana ran into medical personnel who were not fully informed of BRCA issues. When she wanted to get tested for the BRCA mutation, her oncologist was against the idea. Her general doctor had recommended the test after hearing that Alana's grandmother had died of ovarian cancer and that Alana had had breast cancer. But the oncologist disagreed. Alana told me, "I said, 'Doctor, my family doctor sent me to do the BRCA test.' And he just told me, 'I don't know why she did that because you're not Jewish.' . . . After this, the oncologist said, 'Well, it's up to you. If you want to go ahead, do it.'" Then, according to Alana, once he learned that Alana was indeed positive, "He just asked the nurse to call me and tell me to make an appointment with the genetic counselor. That's it. And the genetic counselor told me that she was going to send him an email telling him that, prescribing the breast MRIs every three months."

Alana says this oncologist was "thinking that only Jewish people" could be BRCA positive. "He repeated the same thing to . . . my family physician," she explains. "He said, 'Why? She's not Jewish.'" Alana's family physician eventually called Alana's oncologist and gynecologist and, when both had "no idea about the BRCA test," she told Alana to find other doctors because she was in "bad hands." When doctors know little about the BRCA gene, getting tested—for example, connecting with test providers and genetic counselors or even learning about the test—becomes significantly more difficult for women, and this makes Alana feel "really scared."

This was the case for other women as well: Alison's health-care providers were initially unfamiliar with the BRCA mutation. As a result, she was made to feel alone or, even worse, as if she were a bit of a hypochondriac. Her medical technicians didn't understand why she was getting mammograms at such a young age, and her gynecologist never suggested surveillance as a possible option for her. Jessica describes feeling as if there were a "brotherhood" of doctors who protected each other, ignored her concerns, and brushed her off when she disagreed with their recommendations.

"I Just Don't Think I Was Adequately Prepared": Cynthia's Story

Another issue women faced was that doctors weren't always fully aware of all the consequences and potential side effects of preventive measures. One woman, Nicole, told me she had "all kinds of issues" after her hysterectomy because of changing hormonal levels, says her doctors never alerted this possibility. "It bothers me that information isn't shared," she explains. Like Nicole, after Cynthia had her ovaries removed in her thirties, she was also unprepared for the side effects of the hormonal shifts she experienced.

> I just don't think I was adequately prepared for all the side effects of that. So I had a lot of weight gain. And I had experienced a lot of things. Like, I had a lot of vaginal dryness. Like the morning right after the oophorectomy, and I was like, "Oh my god, what happened?" You know, it's like, "Oh my god, what is going on?" But I feel like it affected my libido a lot, and things like my skin and my fingernails. I just felt like I was changing in ways, slowly, that probably would have happened anyways, but was definitely faster for somebody my age.

So one way medical professionals can help BRCA-positive mutation women make empowering choices is to better inform them about their options. Women should have enough information to make the best decisions for themselves and to be fully aware of the implications of those decisions.

Many women shared these issues of navigating their BRCA journey. There are more problems that were common to many of the women I interviewed. Some women expressed reservations about their doctors' imposition of traditional values and gender role expectations, saying that these unduly influenced surgical decisions. Caitlin was convinced by her doctors to postpone an oophorectomy only when they argued that she should not want to undergo menopause at such a young age. They initially argued that she should want to keep her ovaries in order to have children, which infuriated Caitlin: "I don't care about babies. I don't want cancer." These stories raise questions about how and why doctors influence their patients' decisions based on their own assumptions, which often have little to do with a woman's health. Why should all women have or want to have children?

An often recommended improvement, according to my informants, was for doctors to pay closer attention to a woman's own wishes and ideas about surgical procedures. One woman, reflecting on having her ovaries removed, said her surgeon rushed her into preventive surgery without giving her time to process post–treatment options. According to another woman, doctors were too forceful in their language regarding when and what surgery she should get. They said, "I would not wait; without question, get your ovaries out." Looking back on her decision, she feels that the undue pressure from her doctors may have limited her sense of real choice. If you remember, one woman's gynecologist told her, "You will not turn forty with your ovaries if I am your doctor." These imperious directives, coming as they often do from health professionals considered expert, raise questions about how many degrees of freedom patients feel they have when making personal medical decisions. A few women critique their experience by placing it in the larger context of a medical community that both encourages and benefits from surgeries. In one interview, a woman wondered aloud whether the recent surgical wave is "overkill" but making doctors "very, very rich." She noted that, while her surgery was an "elegant, scientific . . . technically skilled job," each breast cost $100,000.

Women's medical decisions are constrained not only by the information and advice they receive from health-care professionals but also by health-care costs, insurance policies or lack of insurance coverage, and how ably they can negotiate with doctors, insurance company representatives, or other members of the health-care establishment. Cost significantly affects whether women get tested and what they decide to do about a positive result. Several women were afraid to get tested because discovering they were positive for the BRCA mutation might have a bearing on their health insurance. Their insurance rate might increase, they thought. Or perhaps they would have difficulty getting coverage with the preexisting condition of the BRCA mutation. One woman had to fight to get tested and obtain the surgery she felt she needed: "The process took months and months. Everything is about cost. I was told, 'We just don't do hysterectomies for no reason.'" Another woman describes a "really uncomfortable situation" forced on her by her insurance plan. "Do I let them operate on me, or do I go out of network and pay a lot for the surgery with a surgeon I trust? Or do I take another kind of surgery and get implants after all?" Yet another's decision depended on finances and insurance policies more directly: she elected preventive surgery in part because her insurance stopped covering her mammograms.

BRCA-positive mutation women encounter some unique difficulties when negotiating the health-care system. But what, specifically, do BRCA-positive mutation women want health-care providers to know? How can knowledge of the lived experience of these women help improve care and change those things about the medical establishment appear to disempower the women making these important pre- and post–testing decisions?

The Importance of Listening to Women

One critical point: a woman's pre- and post–testing decisions happen in the wide and complicated context of her individual life, and care providers— from genetic counselors to general practitioners to oncologists—must understand this fact. As discussed, doctors and researchers often assume that BRCA-positive mutation women will follow a traditional, rational decision-making model, once they are informed of their genetic risk. However, as we listen to women's stories, we understand that this model does not begin to capture the variety and depth of a woman's decision-making process.

One of the central things BRCA-positive mutation women strive for is to feel in control of their cancer risk. Indeed, many women take up the genetic industry's campaign message that knowledge is power. They believe strongly that they can tackle their cancer risk once they are armed with the information that they do, in fact, harbor the BRCA mutation. In many cases, women think they can eradicate their cancer risk by electing to have surgery.

The stories of these women are complicated, though. Each woman has a personal history and various relationships, and each woman makes unique decisions based on her circumstances. In general, BRCA-positive mutation women do not calculate their risk of getting cancer directly from the statistical data provided by their genetic counselor or physician. Instead, they reframe their risk by filtering the medical odds they are given to reflect a broader nexus of decision making—one that includes their familial history, their firsthand experience of living with relatives who have died from or had cancer, as well as their assessment of the level of social support and information they can draw on from family, friends, and online relationships and networks. Family is particularly important to women's decision-making (Kenan et al. 2007; Koehly et al. 2008). A woman's assessment of her perceived risk and her post–testing medical decisions may have little to do with the medical establishment's presentation of the statistical odds of cancer.

Because so much is involved in a woman's decision-making process and because these choices are often difficult to make, empowerment depends greatly on whether a woman takes control of this process, however it proceeds. Women who feel empowered by their choices often seek out alternative medical information from family and friends, as well as from websites connecting women who are BRCA positive. They often question and exchange ideas with medical providers. And many follow through on their choices in spite of some opposition from others, even taking on the medical profession if they feel strongly that their decisions are right for them. BRCA-positive mutation women frequently regard surgery as an inherently empowering choice, even though some women experience difficult procedures and post–surgical complications. Why should it empower more than, say, surveillance? For one thing, many women trust unwaveringly in the power of preventative surgery to eradicate both their cancer risk and their fear of getting cancer.

Yet whatever decision a woman makes, it can empower her as long as support is available. Genetic counselors and other health-care providers must recognize this larger nexus of decision making and place their recommendations into this context, which is unique for each woman. By analyzing BRCA-positive mutation women's posts on message boards, Kenen and others (2007) made a similar recommendation: "The content of counseling required of health professionals caring for women from HBOC families should be expanded to include the effect of other members of a woman's social world" (Kenen et al. 2007, 796–97).

Genetic counseling should also move to a family-centered model—one that sees a BRCA-positive woman's life as centered within a larger family unit. Although not all women are close to their families, genetic counselors must be aware of the family dynamics involved when women test positive for the BRCA mutation. Counseling is not just about informing a woman about her risk—it must also address the potential familial fallout once she shares her news. How can genetic counseling work with distraught families? What are some strategies for helping women conform to their moral obligation to tell family members about the BRCA mutation while avoiding the family disruptions we have witnessed? Even when a woman expects family support, genetic counselors must give her the tools to deal with the news for herself and weigh post–testing options. Genetic counselors can even offer to invite family members into a counseling session to help facilitate the conversation and explain the implications of one person's positive result on the family.

All health-care providers should consider not only a woman's BRCA-positive mutation status and cancer risk but also her thoughts and feelings. For example, surgeons who perform double mastectomies and oophorectomies need to be aware of the extent to which they harbor gendered stereotypes and to be mindful to avoid imposing their own ideals concerning women's bodies when performing reconstructive surgery. Instead, doctors must listen to what women say about their own needs and preferences with regard to the type of surgery they want and what their ideal surgical outcome might look like. Before even recommending surgery, medical-care providers must give women enough time to process all available options. As well, it is their responsibility to give women comprehensive information about every option. Most important, health-care providers must guide women, but allow them to take responsibility and have a stake in their medical decisions.

Adding New Voices to the Conversation

This book and the wider testing culture for hereditary breast and ovarian cancer have largely left out many who might have the BRCA mutation. Men are not included, nor are marginalized women without the financial or educational resources necessary to consider genetic testing. More individuals will be included and empowered when we recognize that those who are BRCA positive don't form a homogeneous group. They differ by class, race, age, sexual orientation—by the whole spectrum of differences reflective of the larger population. The findings discussed here, as well those of most studies, are based primarily on the experiences of white, middle- to upper-middle-class women. Although I spoke with some women of color, their voices are largely missing from my interviews and from the genetic-testing culture in general, and that must change. This call to broaden inquiry has been echoed in much of the existing social research on BRCA testing (to name a few: Lagos et al. 2008; Mogilner et al. 1998; Sussner et al. 2010). It is imperative that we weave the diversity of women's lived experiences into our understanding of what it means to be a BRCA1- or BRCA2-mutation carrier, especially focusing on marginalized populations (Nelson, Gould, and Keller-Olaman 2009).

Part of this broadening entails an examination of the larger structural issues affecting the medical care of women of color or women living in poverty. How can Hispanic women, black women, Asian women, and more women of color be incorporated into the BRCA conversation? Why doesn't genetic testing reach marginalized communities? The financial issues discussed earlier leave a glaring inequity: BRCA testing and preventive surgeries are often deemed nonessential procedures, leaving women to pay for them out of their own pockets. This type of attitude, finds poor women excluded from the BRCA experience and, potentially, from preventing cancer diagnoses and death. Medicaid and other private and public insurance providers should cover BRCA testing for at-risk individuals as well as the preventive steps, such as surveillance or surgery, that BRCA-positive women subsequently choose.

Racial and cultural issues also have implications for health-care providers, and these sociocultural circumstances can affect the support that women receive in their BRCA journeys. Ethnic, racial, and class differences can complicate a woman's response to her BRCA-positive diagnosis. Perhaps her culture or her religious beliefs encourage fatalism. Or maybe traditional approaches to decision making or to families confuse both her ability to choose and her relations with health care providers. Remember June? Her Chinese immigrant family members pressured her not to get preventative surgery but instead, to accept her fate.

Although men diagnosed with the BRCA mutation are at lower risk for cancer than BRCA-positive women, little attention is paid to the impact of this diagnosis on the lives of these men, which has important implications for both men and women. The BRCA mutation increases men's own risk of breast and prostate cancer (Levy-Lahad and Friedman 2007). Men face some similar decisions when they are diagnosed and, as carriers, they can pass the BRCA mutation on to their offspring. However, the diversity of men's BRCA experiences remains subjugated and just as women begin their process of finding their new normal, especially after undergoing surgery, we know little about the diversity of men's bodily experiences—from deciding to get tested, not getting tested, and/or surveillance and surgical experiences. How do men navigate their gendered identity, and sense of body esteem, especially with regard to how they navigate being masculine especially those who undergo breast and/or prostate surgeries? (Oliffe 2006; Kelly 2009).

My own interviews and other studies reveal that women who inform their male relatives about their risk status find they are often reluctant to get tested or even express hostility about being told (Daly 2009; Strørmsvik et al. 2009). They tend to get tested for the sake of their families and prefer denial in dealing with their own and family members' cancer risk. Although most studies had limited samples, they have suggested that men are reluctant to seek out genetic counseling, which has implications for their own and their families' health. Contrary to how women come together in "BRCA sisterhood," men find it difficult to talk to other men and instead rely on women's support (Strømsvik et al. 2010). Research into health care in general also shows gendered experiences with health care; men are less willing, by and large, to seek out medical treatment for illness or other social support (Daly 2009; Kelly 2009). This finding is not too surprising, given societal definitions of masculinity and the traditional expectation for men to be individualistic and strong. Breast cancer, in particular, carries a social stigma for men, as it is largely associated with women and might be seen as a threat to masculinity. At the same time, men feel guilty about passing on the BRCA mutation to their children. They often seem stuck between their feelings for and against testing (Strørmsvik et al. 2009). Understanding and addressing men's BRCA experience and the masculinity issues associated with being labeled as a BRCA mutation carrier, are important steps in the process of including men and investigating how hereditary breast cancer impacts families as a whole. Some research has shown, for example, that getting back to their new normal, often begins with men seeking to quickly return to their old selves. For some BRCA-positive mutation men, especially those who have had breast and/or prostate cancer, it may mean sticking closely to traditional gendered roles—going to work, trying to "look normal," (even if they can't work), while at the same time, beginning to find their own new normal (Manderson and Peake 2005). Genetic counselors, then, may need to think about taking a different type of counseling approach when addressing men's BRCA experience and breast cancer risk (Daly 2009; Strømsvik et al. 2010).

At the center of this book are the experiences of women as they go through their BRCA-positive journey. However, as we have seen, men—husbands, fathers, brothers, sons, doctors, and other medical caregivers—are often crucial to how women feel about this journey. Does my husband really support my decisions? Will any man be attracted to my post–surgical body? How does my boyfriend really feel about the amount of time I'm spending with my BRCA sisters? What about the amount of money I spent on reconstructive surgery? Is my son really okay with the knowledge that he could have and pass on BRCA1? These questions, often only hinted at, indicate the significant role of men to those who've tested positive for the BRCA mutation. In the interviews, men are often background characters. None-theless, they are important to the women who depend on them and care about them. It is important to widen our lens of understanding by incor-porating the perspective of these significant actors. Knowing, for example, the issues and concerns that a spouse or other close family member voices might enable medical care givers to better treat and counsel not only BRCA-positive women but also those who are directly involved in caring and sup-porting them.

Women in the Testing Culture

This research has uncovered several important policy issues that need to be addressed in order to better serve women dealing with genetic cancer risk. In particular, we must change how women encounter messages from the genetics testing industry and reform how BRCA-positive women are informed of their cancer risk and treatment options. We must ensure that the marketing mes-sages of the genetics testing industry are accurate and sensitive to how testing information is delivered. There needs to be oversight by the FDA regarding quality control of genetic testing procedures to ensure their accuracy.

In chapter 1, I showed how the genetics industry promotes testing for the BRCA mutation, casting a wide net through direct-to-consumer advertis-ing so as to reach as many women as possible. Scores of these women are not at high risk for hereditary cancer. Nonetheless, this testing feeds the health-care industry by promoting preventative surgery. And these "nones-sential" mastectomies, oophorectomies, and hysterectomies happen to be highly lucrative medical procedures. To compound matters, the U.S. medi-cal system privileges consumer choice and urges individuals (who can afford it) to take responsibility for their own health. This orientation often makes women more susceptible to cultural factors, rather than medical advice and counseling, when they choose treatments. So, on one front, the proliferation of direct-to-consumer marketing exposes many women to genetics testing by making it directly available to the consumer, and, on the other, the pre-ventive medical model normalizes genetic testing as part of an individual's prevention regime. The consequence is that more and more women are get-ting tested, but, at the same time, fewer can access medical experts so as to get an accurate interpretation of their genetic testing results. In addition, there appears to be little governmental regulation on the overall reliability and quality of testing procedures. So women can receive false positive or false negative results. The FDA needs to increase efforts to regulate testing procedures and advertisements and to understand the experiences of women and individuals drawn into the testing culture.

Some progress has been made. The Genetic Information Nondiscrimination Act of 2008, which took effect in 2009, protects individuals from being discriminated against by health insurers or employers due to their genetic makeup (National Institutes of Health 2010). This law has made individuals freer to pursue BRCA testing without repercussions and practitioners more willing to recommend testing, as awareness of the law increases (Lowstuter et al. 2008). As Christina admits, "One of the deciding factors in my decision to get tested was the fact that officially genetic discrimination became illegal." She was tested after the law passed.

Another growing area of research and concern is preimplantation genetic diagnosis (PGD), a procedure that looks for genetic disease prior to the implantation of an embryo that is fertilized outside the body. With PGD, a BRCA-positive woman can avoid passing on the BRCA mutation. But the procedure is a source of ethical debate. PGD is especially relevant to women who choose to use in vitro fertilization (IVF) in order to have children after they've undergone a preventive oophorectomy that leaves the uterus in place. A woman would only be able to elect PGD if she also elected, and could afford, IVF, so it is more common among women with coexisting infertility issues (Sagi et al. 2009).

The ethics of using PGD worried many of my interviewees. For example, Isabelle originally supported it: "There is no reason to, you know, have a child with BRCA. If I can prevent this, why would I have my children have the same thing as me?" But, after further consideration, she realized it was not what she wanted because there was a chance that PGD would increase her already high risk of ovarian cancer and because her geneticist advised her that the procedure was not necessary.

> You know, morals aside, religion aside, their professional opinion as doctors is that they don't think PGD is worth it for the BRCA gene because they see so many patients that are okay with the gene and that it's something manageable. . . . You know, I have it, and I'm doing just fine. And my mom is doing just fine. And yes, my aunt died, but we're doing things that, because my aunt gave us knowledge, we can hopefully prevent them. And this is just one thing.

Isabelle is confident that she will have her own children and can raise them knowing they, too, will have to face their cancer risk one day.

Other women see PGD as a way to end the devastating path of the BRCA mutation through the generations. Sam particularly feels this way because she is "the last person in [her] family who has the gene that can have children," so she has the power to "end the whole mutation line." She elaborates:

> If the science is available to do it, I don't see why I wouldn't use it. . . . It doesn't come up a lot within the [FORCE] community just because there are very, very strong feelings about it. Um, but I've read numerous articles, and I've actually talked to someone who had it done. . . . And if I can ensure that, you know, my child, if I choose to have one, would never have to be worried about cancer like I have, why wouldn't I?

Even if Sam herself wouldn't be here if her parents had used PGD, such hypotheticals don't change the fact that Sam would want to prevent any of her children from having to deal with BRCA. Other women are not so sure. One woman who isn't ethically opposed to PGD discussed its ramifications when her daughter considered the procedure: the physical trauma of IVF, the possibility of other health issues not related to BRCA, the expense, the ethics of ending a potential life, and professionals' opinions that the benefits did not outweigh the risks.

Although I was surprised, initially, when this topic surfaced in the interviews, PGD has recently been explored in numerous research studies. Genetic screening is a relatively uncommon procedure, but BRCA-positive mutation women usually see it as an option that should be available (Fortuny et al. 2009; Menon et al. 2007; Ormondroyd et al. 2011; Sagi et al. 2009; Quinn et al. 2010; Vadaparampil et al. 2009). PGD helps women avoid a strong source of guilt and fear—that they will pass the BRCA mutation and its challenges on to their children. Because of their attitudes toward abortion, most women find PGD and embryo selection more acceptable than prenatal diagnosis and terminating a pregnancy (Ormondroyd et al. 2011; Franklin and Roberts 2006). However, ethical issues arise with the idea of pre-designing children. What is the end of the slippery slope of genetic testing before birth? Even though the physical difficulty and expensive of IVF keeps it out of most women's reach, PGD is a growing area for researchers, ethicists, and policy makers to explore.

So what have we learned about how BRCA-positive women would like health care to change? Here is a summary of what these women would recommend.

- Health-care providers (including general practitioners, genetic counselors, and surgeons) must listen to women, answer their questions, and support women's empowered decision-making. Providers need to acknowledge the nexus of decision making in which women process their testing results and make post–testing decisions.
- Counselors should consider following a family-centered approach that acknowledges the broader implications of a positive BRCA result—an approach that extends beyond a single patient and her physical well-being.
- Materials about genetic testing and post–testing options should be clear, informative, and free of medical jargon.
- Health-care providers need to increase their knowledge of genetic testing and hereditary cancer, as well as their ability to communicate testing results and treatment options to women. People should not be left alone, without medical expertise, to interpret test results or make important post–test decisions. In lieu of getting a comprehensive education on these topics themselves, providers should make referrals to other medical professionals.
- Women need to be educated about all post–test options and about all the side effects or consequences of any surgical or surveillance procedures.
- Insurance companies must not allow BRCA status to affect a woman's coverage; policies should also cover testing for at-risk women, as well as preventive surgery or surveillance procedures for those who test positive.

Research on the experiences of BRCA-positive mutation women has led to numerous similar recommendations from other scholars, such as targeting recruitment materials for BRCA testing to culturally and ethnically diverse men and women (Daly 2009; Vadaparampil and Pal 2010); recognizing the broad context of women's decision-making (Howard et al. 2010); and providing multitiered professional- and peer-led support for BRCA-positive individuals, including websites and online chat forums, workshops, social events, phone lines, and newsletters (Hughes and Phelps 2010; Lloyd et al. 2000). Provider education must improve as well. Currently, women receive widely different recommendations for risk management, ones that stray from the National Comprehensive Cancer Network's guidelines. This confusion often leaves women not knowing about their options for screening or surgery (Dhar et al. 2011). Research also recommends that all post–testing options be discussed at the time of testing, before women get the results, so they are prepared if and when they get a positive one (Lloyd et al. 2000; Mahon 2011). Scholars also affirm the need for counselors to discuss social support and the quality of a patient's relationships, as well as giving their clients full descriptions of surgical procedures.

Finding Empowerment: Revisiting June's Story

> I'm overall a pretty strong-minded person. If I want something, I want to get it over with and get it done. I'm not one of those like, wishy-washy. It just has to be the right timing, and being in the right atmosphere.

June has proved to be an extremely determined woman. One and a half years after our first conversation, June's story revisited me when I received an e-mail from her, updating me on her life and medical development. She told me she moved out from her parents' house, bought her own home, and flew to Europe for six months to have her breasts removed, without telling any of her friends, coworkers, or family members! I was shocked and hopeful at this turnaround of events in her life.

Some women do find a sense of empowerment throughout their BRCA experience, although this process may take many years. When I first met June, she was stuck in surveillance, unsure how she might proceed from surveillance to surgery, without familial support and medical guidance. Now, in conversation with her, June radiated extreme confidence, exhibiting the characteristics of a woman who has determinedly seized the opportunities before her. When a close friend explained that June could benefit from the dismal housing market, June, in her own words, "went for it": she moved out from her parents' house and bought her own home. June explains that "things started happening in my direction, when I was able to acquire my own place," and this gave her previously unheard of degree of adulthood and independence. June now feels that "Having my own home, my own private space, I can do whatever I want. I didn't have to worry about what others think." This new sense of empowerment and autonomy further impelled

June to go to Europe to have a double mastectomy: "So, then I went for it, and I said, "Okay." . . . that's when I decided to take time off and go to Europe and have my surgeries." This was the next leg of June's road to empowerment.

June's choice to travel to Europe was a bold one: she was still untested for BRCA at the time, and she did not tell anyone her real reason for traveling. Instead, she told her family and friends she was going on a sabbatical. This reveals June's striking determination to address her cancer head-on, a striking change from how stuck she previously felt in surveillance. June explains this as a strong choice that emanated from her newfound separation from her parents' dissenting opinions over her medical decision making.

> Once I found out that you know, having the breast cancer gene, I knew it was coming one day . . . I mean, yeah, I could be making the biggest mistake of my life, I may never have cancer, you know? . . . But I'd rather . . . get it over with than to have to deal with it, you know? . . . But it's just that, as long as I'm still under my parents' house, under their roof, I can't do anything like that. I can't have my own privacy.

June's newfound independence allowed her to move out of living with her parents and to buy her own home. Furthermore, it provides June with the impetus to "get it [having her surgeries] over with" and moving on toward her new normal, rather than waiting for cancer to come. June explains that her move out was a motivator for getting "unstuck."

Her decision to fly to Europe to cross over into surgery reveals a determination to live her own life. June explains that she did not like the American hospitals because they did not exude the same vitality she felt in spite of her cancer.

> I wasn't ready to do it in the U.S., because I visited the hospitals, and the choices . . . It just didn't felt like something I want, you know? I'm not sick . . . I see it as more like an elective surgery. I'm not dying yet . . . So, I don't want to be in an environment where people are so sad.

June held an upbeat attitude toward BRCA and cancer throughout her procedures. She felt that she was not a cancerous patient, but instead was someone being practical and proactive about her health. Rather than fighting it, June was able to accept her BRCA-positive diagnosis as simply a "confirmation" of what she already knew, because this whole process was "inevitable." June felt strong in her decisions that this was simply a stage of her life, one that she will pass through and move on from into her new normal.

In a compelling reversal from her prior insecurities over her body and her breasts, June now feels very confident in her new body post-surgery. She told me that her surgeons "did a good job" with her double mastectomy, and that her breasts were healing well. She explained calmly how "I see the line across of me, you know, on each one of my breasts where they were. Because it's just flat now. That, that hill is gone. So, so they literally removed from side to side." Her unemotional explanation of the loss of her breasts illustrates how, unlike much of prevalent culture, she does not consider women's breasts a sexual or sexualized part of the body. Her breasts are not integral to her own identity. June explained that unlike other women who have emotional attachments to their breasts, especially in their identification as women, that, "I don't have of that kind of feeling for my breasts going away." June explained this for me further.

> Having no breasts is just very, very, I could say, call it very, materialistic, you know, in a way. . . . Because, it's just an extra. Before, a woman used to say, "That defines us." . . . I mean, I feel like it's degrading when you say, you know, I know it's the norm that women are supposed to have breasts. But it's just that, I think over the years because this breast image thing that is so important, that a woman must have. It's more like degrading a woman, you know? Cause what happened, whatever happened to the good old days when the breasts is not even a sexual toy? It's a mechanism to feed the young ones, if you had a baby, you know? So it's just there for that. It's for a useful purpose. It's not, not as a sexual object to please a guy. So I'm not, I'm not at all upset without, with no breasts.

While before June struggled to reconcile not being the "ideal of the petite Chinese girl," now she feels very confident in her body image, explaining to me that "I kinda enjoy being fat." In fact, she responded a resounding "Yeah!" when I asked her, "Do you feel okay about how you look?" This is why June decided against any reconstruction: to prevent any possibility of cancer and because she did not find it necessary to her identity as a woman.

As June continues to move forward, however, one thing that has not changed is her lack of a strong support network. June's loneliness has not changed since we last spoke, and she has become even more estranged from her family, further alienating her from the familial support I found to be so crucial for other women on this journey. June still has very few people to rely on. She has not told her family at all about her surgeries or her BRCA-positive mutation result, telling me that "I probably will keep [my results and surgeries] to myself. They don't wanna hear about it, you know. I don't wanna deal with it, cause I would just be opening a new can of worms for myself." Yet June remains concerned for her family, explaining that she is "hoping that nobody else in the family will carry" the gene. But after her long struggle over her medical choices, June has resigned herself to the fact that if her sister does ultimately have the BRCA gene or cancer, that "it's already her choice. I've already mentioned it to her. She's an adult, I can't force her to go get tested." In fact, June admits that her parents may never be ready to know about the real reason for her trip to Europe: "I'm just hoping that I won't have to tell them, you know? But I mean, maybe years and years from now. . . ."

Yet, what June does not articulate is truly how alienating this is. The previous chapters have exemplified how much a woman's network of support—wherever she finds it—is crucial to her physical, mental, and emotional well-being in every step of the BRCA mutation decision-making process. With her family's lack of support, her coworkers' ignorance, and the little involvement of few friends, June still struggles to find a source of support and inspiration throughout her decision making. Thus, June still clings to celebrities and the media for guidance. June explained this influence upon her medical decision making.

> Rich people, I always hear it on TV . . . that they go to rich spas, and stuff like that . . . So then I said, "Hmm. . . . Is that possible?" That's when I started emailing the clinic over there. And they actually wrote back, so, you know, and that's how it all got connected. Cause I wasn't going, I was thinking, "There has to be a way. The rich wanted all that privacy," you know? They're not gonna be, you know, someone so famous, they're not gonna be shown checking into the local hospital for treatment or something.

With a lack of better role models, June chose to emulate celebrities in many realms of decision making: the possibility of adopting children, medical choices, and friendships within the BRCA community. June feels a common link between herself and the celebrities she sees on TV, and she uses them as role models due to a lack of similar support in her immediate life—namely, the more common support network of close family members, significant others, or friends.

June continues to look optimistically to the future, however. She is considering removing her ovaries in addition to her breast, but she explained that she is currently on a "five-year plan" in order to meet a man who could be both a life partner and a father. Since our first interview, she has come far in her initial fear of finding a partner who would respect her decisions and her surgeries, and support and love her despite being BRCA positive. This empowerment radiated throughout our conversation, as she explained her refusal to let her removed breasts become a problem in dating.

> I know for sure, I will not undergo reconstruction just for a guy. I'm not willing to do that. I'm not. I want him to like me for who I am. So what if I have no breasts, no nipples. He's gonna have to accept me the way I am, you know? If he cannot, then I guess he's not the right guy.

This reveals a new, strong sense of self as part of June's overall journey toward her new normal and personal empowerment.

During our initial interview, June felt disempowered and stuck in the surveillance category of waiting for cancer to come. Now, however, she lives a very different story. While June continues to struggle in finding a support network, she no longer lives with her parents, whom she considered detrimental to her health. Instead, she owns her own home and is making strong choices for herself in many realms of her health and her life. June's new normal is radically different from what it was before, but she has emerged from this multiyear journey to a new sense of independence and personal empowerment.

Concluding Reflections

One way to picture the pathways women take in their BRCA journey is to imagine a spiral that circles back to a new beginning but continues to move through the generations. Or, as one woman puts it, "Cancer runs through my family like water through a sieve." Some women have already heard different generation's narratives about waiting for cancer to come. These tales are shared among family members—as warnings, encouragements, or messages of hope. In other families, stories are untold or hidden until cancer strikes and brings the revelation that the disease runs through the family tree.

The one-size-fits-all thinking about patients that places them into diagnostic boxes does not fully address women's needs, concerns, and values. The medical community must recognize that patients never follow the exact same pathway of decision-making; that each person's journey, as we have observed, is embedded in the wider context of relationships and experiences, and especially within the history of cancer in that individual's family. A woman, when she searches for her own way through the BRCA experience, often traces the journey of a relative who has gone before. She especially chooses when to get tested, and if or when to get surgery, based on the "cancer clocks" of her family members who have already been diagnosed. BRCA-positive mutation women carefully calibrate how much time they may have to wait before cancer comes, and, while they wait, they plan for the future, although they're painfully aware of the risk of cancer lurking in the background.

Although some women's pathways are already mapped for them, others find themselves alone on this journey with no family history to guide them. At what age should I get tested? When should I get surgery and what type? Each of these women must come to independent answers. These women are pioneers; they are charting new territory for their families. Some may turn more to websites to gain perspective on what lies ahead, listening to the stories of women who are outside their bloodlines but become their BRCA sisters. Many women decide to make the journey together with a close relative, sisters joining sisters, a mother uniting with her daughters, or an aunt with her niece.

When we listen deeply to BRCA-positive mutation women's stories, we realize how their actions are so often shaped by their experiences and connections to others. Getting tested, taking preventative steps, and a host of other decisions are taken from amidst a woman's daily connections to family, friends, and other people in her life. These decisions are also embedded in the values of the racial and ethnic cultures each woman grew up in and in the economic conditions under which each lives out her life. Women's decisions are also increasingly shaped by larger environmental factors, such as our culture moving toward the normalization of genetic testing and cancer prevention—a trend that brings even more women into the testing culture, even those at very low risk for genetic disorders.

Whatever statistics, health-care providers, researchers, or medical guidelines might say, each woman's experience is different, and it is only by empowering each woman and supporting her as an individual that we can uplift women and allow them to live healthy and fulfilling lives. Moving toward a better understanding of how to provide care for each woman and all women who have the BRCA hereditary mutation requires an approach by researchers, health-care professionals, communities, and our culture that centers on women's experiences and concerns. Statistics are one thing. They tell only part of the story, and, for many women, not a very significant part. More important than medical models of risk assessment, or preventative measures that give the best odds of never having to hear the feared words "you have cancer," are policies that empower women to make whatever decisions are best for them. And we mean all women, not just wealthy ones.

So how do we frame these policies? Inform women fully. And listen to them carefully. Consider each as a unique individual within a specific context when giving advice. Develop measures that enable the women who are most at risk, women from all walks of life, to get the information and medical procedures they need to maintain not only their lives but also the quality of those lives. It is these sets of questions and their answers that will serve to guide an empowering set of pathways for women whose lives cross paths with the BRCA mutation.

Epilogue

Through Their Eyes:
Studying Women's Health

Waiting for Cancer to Come is a book about the experiences of women who have tested positive for the BRCA1 and BRCA2 gene mutations that indicate increased risk of breast and ovarian cancer. This book grew out of a research project that sought to explore the lived experiences of such women. I was fortunate enough to investigate this topic through the eyes of engaged and passionate women who honored me by sharing their stories. Through our conversations, I delved deeper into their motivations for getting tested, the roles played by their families and others important in their lives, the decisions they made post-testing, and other events and circumstances significant to their BRCA journeys.

As a professor of sociology and director of the Women's and Gender Studies Program at Boston College, I have researched a variety of topics related to women's lives and health, including women and work, the intersection of gender and race, and body image and eating disorders. In my work, I strive to uplift the voices of women whose knowledge has been subjugated and is often missing in other scholars' work, as well as to use my research to better women's lives. And as you saw in the prologue, more personal reasons first inspired me to explore the issues women deal with when diagnosed with breast and ovarian cancer. Once I was tested for the BRCA mutation gene myself and reflected more on the proliferation of genetic testing in general, I was drawn to this topic. Because of my personal experiences and my academic background in feminist research, this study found me.

Where Are Women's Voices?

As I first began to explore the BRCA experience in the medical literature, I realized that I wasn't hearing women's voices in terms of their experiences with genetic testing and their post–testing medical decision making. Although a valuable body of research is available in the burgeoning field of genetic testing and testing for hereditary breast and ovarian cancer in particular, few researchers allowed women to drive the research by telling their stories and revealing new and unexpected areas to explore.

Feminist scholars have done work in the area of genetics with regard to prenatal diagnosis, as well as the ethical and social implications of new reproductive technologies such as preimplantation genetic diagnosis (Shaffer and den Veyver 2012; Rothman 1998; Steinberg 1997). There is little research on the overall lived experiences of women who undergo genetic testing for the BRCA1 and 2 gene mutations, especially related to how BRCA-positive women assess their risk for developing cancer (Finkler, Skrzynia, and Evans 2003; Hamilton et al. 2009; Mellon et al. 2009; Salant et al. 2006; Sorenson and Botkin 2003).

Some research studies that focus specifically on BRCA-positive mutation women's assessment of their cancer risk reveal that they have trouble understanding the probability of their cancer risk their physicians and genetic counselors present to them (Brown et al. 2011; Kenen, Arden-Jones, and Eeles 2003; Portnoy, Roter, and Erby 2010). Zikmund-Fisher, Fagerlin, and Ubel (2010) argue that the way medical personnel currently deliver this risk information is insensitive to the emotional state and the cognitive understanding of their clients. They should calibrate their delivery of this information by not only thinking "what risk information [they] want [their] audience to think about" but also "what feelings will this message evoke?" and how they can be more understanding to these sentiments that arise from this difficult and confusing news (7).

Much of the research literature on medical decision making assumes that women who test positive for the BRCA mutation will follow a specific decision-making protocol. This literature assumes that women adhere to their care providers' expert knowledge and decide on a course of action based on a self-described rational medical decision-making model (Rodney et al. 2004). Many medical personnel assume that once women know about their risk, these women can be "managed" and they should "comply" with their recommendations, and a lot of emphasis is given on identifying at-risk women with the assumption that once they are identified, their care can be made more efficient and effective (Pilarski 2009, 305; Ozanne et al. 2009).

Yet research on how women actually evaluate their risk and treatment choices is under-researched, which questions the validity and actuality of such assumptions (Hopwood et al. 2000; Lerman et al. 2000; Metcalfe and Narod 2002). Some research suggests that women tend to inflate their actual objective risk (for reasons discussed throughout this book, such as identifying one's risk by her mother's cancer clock). Indeed, a research study of women with a familial history of breast cancer found that individual risk assessment was experienced through the lens of their family's experience with cancer, often resulting in heightened fear and vulnerability (Chalmers and Thompson 1996). This often pushes women to pursue inappropriate or unnecessary risky preventative surgeries (Heshka et al. 2008; Sivell et al. 2008; d'Agincouirt-Canning 2005; Hallowell et al. 2001).

In much of this prior research noted earlier, I found strong parallels between the experiences of the women it described, and in the stories of the women I spoke with. Simultaneously, however, I found several areas lacking the necessary depth to adequately discuss this topic, and this allowed me to draw my own conclusions. Some of these conjectures differed from existing material, and this pushed me to provide my own recommendations on improving women's BRCA testing, surveillance, and surgical experiences. This absence of women's lived experiences of breast and ovarian cancer risk assessment, genetic testing, and subsequent medical decision making pushed me further into conducting my own project to truly incorporate women's voices into this discussion. The incorporation of the feminist standpoint methodology is crucial to doing so.

A Feminist Standpoint Approach
to the BRCA-Positive Mutation Experience

The theoretical lens I take onto this research project is that of a feminist standpoint approach, which builds knowledge through women's lived experiences and unearths subjugated knowledge within this epistemology that otherwise would remain hidden and unanalyzed. Dorothy Smith (1987) and Sandra Harding (1987) were early proponents of the standpoint perspective that stresses the necessity of women's everyday experiences. Through analyzing the gaps between the perspectives of women's real lived experiences and the dominant culture's conceptualization such as that of the dominant medical paradigm of risk assessment, the researcher gains a more accurate and theoretically richer set of explanations of the lives of women, as well as a better understanding of hegemonic groups and cultures (Hesse-Biber 2007,

2012). This concept of multiple vantage points has been further incorporated into later versions of standpoint theory, by stressing the importance of the interlocking relationships between racism, sexism, heterosexism, and class oppression as additional starting points into understanding women's social realities (Harding 1987; Collins 1990; Mohanty 1988; hooks 1984; Anzaldu'a 1987). Still other feminist researchers such as Haraway (1988) cautioned against privileging any given standpoint as the "most oppressive" or the "most valid," because this would lead to hierarchically valuing some perspectives as "better" or "truer" than others, which discounts women's experiences overall. I found Donna Haraway's concept of "situated knowledges" (1988)—the particular social locations of individuals as an important starting point for understanding subjective experience—particularly relevant in getting at women's lived experiences in my own work.

A feminist standpoint approach to knowledge building praxis consists of deeply listening to accounts of women's *experiences*, specifically concerning how they understand the role that genetic testing has played in their lives, and how they come to understand their cancer risk and treatment options. In taking a feminist standpoint approach, we argue that it is only by taking into account women's subjective experience in assessing their genetic risk, that one can reveal the subjugated knowledge of our own understanding of women's risk assessment, and incorporate it into a conceptualization that intersects with the standard medical model of assessing cancer risk.

Through the feminist standpoint approach, our qualitative data analysis looks at the decision-making calculus women employ as they grapple with what to do after testing positive for the BRCA mutation. Their decision-making nexus involves a range of engagements with medical caregivers as well as family and close friends. Our findings reveal that the decision-making process is highly complex, iterative, and subject to reassessment over time, as women reach out to their social, medical, and online networks to both learn more about their medical condition and to listen to other women's stories of being BRCA positive. Women also explore their family's cancer history in depth as a way to calculate their risk for getting cancer and use that to weigh treatment options provided by care providers (oncologists and/or genetics counselors).

Because of this range and the subsequent variety of women's experiences, I set out with no specific hypothesis that I sought to test, and I did not have this book or even a particular article in mind. As I designed my project and began to speak with individual women, I remained as open as possible to allow what the women I interviewed defined as the most important to rise to the surface. The research design helped me to remain open and prioritize the voices of the women I spoke with in each stage of the research process.

The process of writing this book—interviewing and surveying women and analyzing their stories—was an intense and profound experience. And that experience, especially the rewards and challenges of speaking with women about such an important and personal topic, is worthy of description.

The Research Project

The Sample

The research study that serves as the basis of this book began with in-depth interviews of sixty-four women, and all of these women tested positive for the BRCA1 or BRCA2 gene mutation except one. I interviewed this woman, who had not gotten the test at the time of our interview, because she elected preventive surgery based on her family history. She was sure, even without the test, that she was positive for the BRCA mutation. (Hers was a unique case that mirrors, in many ways, the experience of actually being a BRCA-positive mutation carrier.)

The women in my study were an average of thirty-nine years old, yet their ages ranged from twenty-three to sixty-six. All were living in the United States. They were predominately Caucasian, middle class, and had completed at least some college. They were fairly diverse by religion: 42 percent Christian, 30 percent Jewish, 7 percent agnostic or atheist, 4 percent Mormon, and 18 percent other or nonreligious. The percentage of Jewish women in the study was disproportionately high compared to national statistics, most likely because of the increased likelihood of Ashkenazi Jews being BRCA carriers. Of the sample, 67 percent of the women were married at the time of the interview, and 52 percent had at least one child; 19 percent had also tested positive for cancer.

The sample of women I interviewed reflects the demographics of women who are generally tested for the BRCA mutation in the United States: white, middle to upper class, and educated with access to the Internet and other information and resources. However, the sample does not reflect the general population and leaves out the multiple and crucial voices of people of color and others who may still be tested but in smaller numbers. The same interlocking factors of inequality, lack of research, and subjugated knowledge that intersect in the genetic testing industry also affected my ability to draw diverse women to my study. In this way, the stories and conclusions I make in this book are not necessarily applicable to women in general or to particular women not represented by my respondents.

Data Collection Methods:
Finding BRCA-Positive Mutation Women

I obtained approval from the Institutional Review Board (IRB) at my college to conduct the research project and followed a strict research protocol that included obtaining women's written consent to be interviewed, as well as their consent to have me record the interview digitally. All real names have been changed in this book to protect the women's identities, and specific identifying information has also been removed or changed to maintain confidentiality. I conducted all of the sixty-four in-depth interviews for this study. I listened to all of the digitized recordings on the average at least twice and was able to write descriptive summaries and analytical memos on the fly. This was done in an iterative fashion whereby each interview was summarized, memos were taken, and some grounded theory coding was conducted before going on to conduct another interview. Research assistants were responsible for transcribing the interviews using HyperTranscribe (www. researchware.com), a computer software transcription program. I then went over each transcript listening for any missing material and to ensure that each interview was fully transcribed, including noting those areas where a respondent would express a strong emotion such as laughter, sadness, and crying. I emailed each respondent her transcription with all her identifying information removed, and I gave each respondent a unique identification number. I only emailed respondents' their transcribed interview if they noted they would like a copy. I suggested that if they did read it over and wanted to change something they said or add any new remarks or material, they should do so and send the interview back to me with any corrections, additions and deletions, and so on.

Participants in this study were selected from women who responded to online research postings I placed in online informative websites to assist post–testing medical decision making, and that encourage BRCA-positive mutation women to share their experiences about being tested. First and foremost, these websites seek to reach out to these women with support as they proceed to come to terms with being a BRCA-mutation gene carrier.

Prior to the interviewing process, I sent each respondent a letter of consent to sign in order to participate in the interview, and each woman was made aware of the confidential nature of the interview process, and that they could terminate the interview at any time. These interviews consisted of open-ended questions, and I recorded them over the telephone. Each woman spoke with me for about one and a half to two hours, talking about their families, the emotions and challenges involved with making decisions about testing and surgery, and anything else they thought was important in defining the BRCA-positive mutation experiences. As this book shows, these women's stories are highly diverse, but they also share some common elements. Many of the women had a very strong history of cancer in their families and had the experience of a blood relative either being diagnosed with a BRCA-related hereditary cancer or dying from cancer. They often knew from a young age that they might be at high risk for cancer, but they waited until they were older to deal with this information.

The Research Design

As a feminist interviewer, I was interested in getting at what is often referred to as *unarticulated knowledge.* My goal was to explore issues of particular concern to BRCA-positive mutation women from their perspective. In developing the study, I kept in mind the various criteria for the quality and validity of qualitative research laid out by Lincoln (1995), including acknowledging the researcher's standpoint, engaging in critical reflexivity, and establishing reciprocity between the researchers and the researched. I also followed up each interview with a survey that allowed me to compare and contrast important demographic information. Sometimes during the interviews, I would share my own hunches of their experiences that I had begun to formulate from the grounded theory analysis along the way—my way of testing these ideas with my respondents.

In each interview, I focused on the nature of my interactions within the interview situation, being mindful of how my particular personal and researcher standpoint entered into the ongoing interview. I paid particular attention to the ways in which my role may have exerted power and author-ity over the interview situation. For example, I considered whether I may have only listened to what I thought was important or asked only those questions that I was particularly interested in asking. In other words, I was aware of the possibility that I would produce knowledge more reflective of my own values and interests (agenda) than those of my respondents.

In order to be mindful of how inequities can arise between the researcher and researched, I was mindful to practice reflexivity concerning what values and attitudes I brought to the research setting. Reflexivity means taking a critical look inward—reflecting on one's own lived reality and experiences. How does your own biography impact the research process? What in your own experience shapes the questions you choose to study and the approach to studying them? How does the specific social, economic, and political context in which you reside affect the research process at all levels? Reflexivity is the process through which a researcher recognizes, examines, and comes to understand how his or her social background and assumptions can intervene in the research process. The researcher is a product of society and its structures and institutions just as much as the researched. Our beliefs, backgrounds, and feelings are part of the process of knowledge construction (Hesse-Biber and Piatelli 2012). To practice reflexivity means to acknowledge, "All knowledge is affected by the social conditions under which it is produced and that it is grounded in both the social location and the social biography of the observer and the observed" (Mann and Kelley 1997, 392).

But these reflexive moments are hard to document. They happen at odd moments and throughout a research project. In my researcher account that follows, I provide an account of the reflexive moments during the project that helped me to place in check my own values, attitudes, and research assumptions. This account shows that conducting research is not a clear-cut, linear, and predictable process. It also demonstrates that researchers who present their work as if nothing crops up in their projects to bias their findings miss an important opportunity to gain more understanding of their own research role that may unwittingly contribute to a range of biases in their research project. Although my training as a researcher provided me with a wealth of skills going into this project, my personal experiences with breast cancer and BRCA testing was so intertwined with my motivations to conduct this study that sharing my reflexive process is essential to reflect on.

In continuing the reflexive process when writing this book, I decided to present my own story in the prologue and at various other points. Scholars increasingly recognize that "story is central to human understanding" (Lewis 2011, 505). My experience with breast cancer and BRCA testing was so intertwined with my research that, on a number of topics, I felt I needed to share my story with you, the readers. As Patrick Lewis (2011) notes, "This more-ness takes us beyond self, to being present with the other . . . and through subsequent storying and reflection, we make small discoveries and beyond those discoveries, in the shadows, we find there is something else, something more" (509).

By the end of the project, I had conducted in-depth interviews with sixty-four women. One respondent's data had to be deleted because the recording of her interview was faulty. Instead of using a fixed set of questions in the interview, I wanted each woman to define what the research agenda would be. Although I wanted to know about different aspects of their BRCA experience very broadly—for example, how they came to be tested for the BRCA mutation and what post–testing decisions they made—I saw my role as listening deeply to their story. The interview took on the form of a narrative. I would start off with a general question: can you tell me how you came to be tested for the BRCA mutation? I usually held off getting extensive demographic data from them, and I only asked them at first a few general demographic questions such as their age, marital status, whether or not they had children, and their occupational status. Not dwelling on getting specific answers allowed me to move away from the survey mode of interviewing, to listen carefully, and to set a more conversational tone.

The Addition of the Online Survey

At the end of each in-depth interview, I asked women whether or not I might contact them again with an online survey that had additional questions related to their interview. All the women agreed that they would be interested in filling out a survey. I restricted the survey sample to the women I had interviewed in order to be able to validate some of my findings from the in-depth interviews with data from the survey. Fifty-six of the women I interviewed—89 percent—completed the survey. The survey covered demographic information such as age and race; information about BRCA testing, personal cancer history, and family history; and more detailed questions to get at women's feelings about being tested and about other steps, such as making decisions based on test results. It also included demographic information including marital status, occupation, education, race, religion, and socioeconomic status. Additional information was taken, where possible, from the interviews of those missing from surveys in order to complete the quantitative data set.

The data derived from the online survey supported in terms of validating the larger themes that women themselves identified in their in-depth interviews that were developed through a grounded theory analysis. For example, I asked women on the survey to estimate how much at risk they felt they were for getting cancer after they received their BRCA-positive result. These answers helped to validate the remarks women made in their interviews with regard to the high degree of fear they felt. The online survey data also supported findings from the interviews about the small time gap these women experienced between being BRCA-positive mutation status and getting cancer. I also asked women about the importance of specific factors that may have encouraged or discouraged them from testing. Those factors that came out as most important in the survey were the same factors that were present in their interviews.

Data Analysis: Using Multiple Analytical Lenses to Understand Women's Experiences

I employed three different types of analytical perspectives as an analytical strategy to uncover the experiences of BRCA-positive mutation women, and each type served to reveal different aspects of these experiences or looked at them in a different way. The first form of analysis I used, poetry, was for me the most personally and unexpectedly valuable one.

The prologue of this book opens with a poetic reflection composed from the voices of these very women. The poem covers a wide range of themes from the interviews, with each line representing a different aspect of one particular woman's experience of being a positive BRCA-mutation carrier. This unusual form of analysis was not planned. It sprang naturally from my response to the stories. Through the data collection and analysis processes, I had a habit of listening to the interview recordings in order to better retain them in my memory. I also felt that hearing the interviews before I went to bed might spark some new analytical and interpretive insights. I wanted to continue to play these recordings in order to hear the tone and silences contained in women's stories, important conversational clues that I might miss by only reading a transcription of interviews. I also felt that playing back the audio recordings helped me find a slightly different angle of understanding, an immediate and intuitive way into my respondents' experiences.

One night, I fell asleep with the recordings still playing. I vividly remember waking from a very deep sleep and still hearing the voices of the women I had interviewed. They were talking with me and with one another about their BRCA-positive mutation related experiences. I immediately recorded what I remembered hearing. These voices became the poem that begins this book. Poetry, I believe, is an important medium for placing women's voices in conversation and dialogue with one another. Through it, I realized that the women's stories revealed an underlying theme of waiting for cancer to come. These voices also revealed how engaged women were in a battle for their lives. They use various military metaphors to describe how they feel under siege by their cancer diagnosis—or by the knowledge that they have the BRCA mutation. The overall tenor of their combined voices conveyed a deep fear, a dread of the future. So many women are at risk and waiting for cancer to come, convinced that it will, and suspended between being cancer-free and feeling that it's just around the corner.

The poem also showcases women's voices in a creative way. Carroll, Dew, and Howden-Chapman (2011) use a similar strategy in their study of people in Aotearoa, New Zealand, living in informal dwellings. In that research, participants' own words form coherent and thematic poetry that captures their experiences. As Caroll, Dew, and Howden-Chapman (2011) argue, "Combining thematic analysis and poetic representation . . . allows for a broader understanding of a phenomenon under investigation. . . . We would also suggest that, for some kinds of knowledge generation and knowledge transfer, poetry may be preferable to conventional social science writing" (628).

The second analysis method I employed was grounded theory analysis, in order to discern underlying patterns of women's experiences within and across interviews (Bryant and Charmaz 2007; Glaser and Strauss 1967; Strauss and Corbin 2000). This method begins with the researcher listening to the interviews and going over the transcriptions line by line. These techniques provide the researcher with a systematic way to derive meaning based on a careful listening to the data, while limiting the influence of researcher bias. Each interview was iteratively analyzed, because this type of in-depth procedure is best for capturing the range of feelings and attitudes of a given respondent, and it allowed these women to talk more openly about their perspective on relevant issues and factors (Charmaz 2006; Hesse-Biber 2007). So my task was to listen to women and capture how they have come to understand their BRCA related experiences and to make the important decisions necessary because of their positive diagnosis (Glaser and Strauss 1967; Strauss and Corbin 2000). Grounded theory analysis allows for the uncovering of women's patterns of behaviors throughout the multitude of voices, such as the extent to which family and friends play a part in genetic testing decisions, how professional and family life plans change as a result of a positive diagnosis, how body-image perceptions changed after testing or surgery, and the extent to which these women's experiences were perceived as empowering or disempowering in their everyday lives.

The coding process is multidimensional, consisting of creating a series of memos and conducting open coding, which is a way of "naming segments of data with a label that simultaneously categorizes, summarizes, and accounts for each piece of data" (Charmaz 2006, 43). This naming process is the beginning of interpretation: what is the data saying? Initial coding may often consist of using descriptive terms that help identify where in the interview the respondent is talking about a certain topic. For example, the code "testing experience" is a descriptive code and comes directly from what is said. This code tells you where in the interview the respondent talks about this topic, but the label does not necessarily reflect an understanding of the process whereby women come to get tested or how they experience that decision. The code, however, provides researchers a means to return to the data and look for the underlying dimensions of the testing situation.

Coding an interview then moves from a descriptive level to a more analytic level to get at these deeper understandings. So, for example, under the code "testing experience" I derived the analytical code "not ready," a theme that emerged from rereading the interview portions related to women's testing experiences. This code is also an "in vivo code," which uses the words of a respondent as a code and comes from carefully listening to the data. Women repeatedly indicated that they spent a period of time where they were "not ready" to get tested. Being ready itself consists of a variety of dimensions, and I teased out of this analytical code a set of "ready dimensions" and factors to describe what contributed to a woman being ready.

Another important aspect of analysis is to discern how various analytical codes relate to one another, a process known as *axial coding*. This step uncovers connections and processes within the data and develops even further codes to reflect these connections. I asked questions like these: How is the code "not ready" related a respondent's family history of cancer? How is it related to each woman's life stage? These axial coding questions might develop other codes, for example, "not ready: no close relative with cancer" or "ready: finished child-bearing years." Connecting codes to one another is also a way to generate a larger theoretical understanding of the processes that comprise women's experience of being BRCA positive.

The third form of analysis I used to analyze and interpret the data was identifying case studies. I found core case studies for the chapters' topics; cases that best exemplified some of the fundamental issues faced by BRCA-positive mutation women. I wanted to retain the integrity of some of the women's stories, so I presented each of these narratives as a whole. Creating case studies allows the reader to observe the process by which specific themes identified by the grounded theory and poetic approach are intertwined and embodied within a given woman's BRCA experience. I chose case studies that reflected a number of the issues and themes discussed in a given chapter. Around each core case study, I also presented a set of shorter cases that reflect experiences different from those represented in the main case. These provide a sense of how individual women's experiences vary.

Reflecting on My Own Research Standpoint

My decision to write this book was a step toward acknowledging my own cancer diagnosis and the history of cancer experiences among my siblings. It was also a way for me to honor the memory of my younger sister and her courage in facing stage IV breast cancer. Over the course of the past three years in which I interviewed women for this book, I found that talking and listening to women about their BRCA testing and post–testing decisions empowered me to move beyond denial of my cancer diagnosis. I, too, was able to begin the process of moving on to my own new normal.

Before I began this research project, I was diagnosed with breast cancer twice over the course of the past ten years. Three years ago, I had breast conserving surgery and radiation therapy. I went out of my way to keep my cancer diagnosis and treatment hidden from others, except for my immediate family. I did not want to take on a somatic identity of being a breast cancer survivor. I did not feel connected to those who embraced a "pink ribbon" breast cancer culture. I resonated with the concerns Barbara Ehrenreich, a feminist journalist and political activist expressed with regard to her own feelings about this community, referring to it as "the pink-ribbon breast cancer cult," whereby women who have cancer are encouraged to join in a sisterhood, that, among other things, requires them to be upbeat and encouraging them to "smile"; that is, "cancer is a gift" (Ehrenreich 2010; Sulik 2010); meaning that having cancer can allow one to reflect on the positive outcomes of having a cancer diagnosis, such as they realize how many friends they have who have come to their aid. This is something I discuss further later on.

Beyond these issues and concerns, what was at the front of my ongoing angst in conducting this study is that I also felt that overtly acknowledging my history of cancer would always remind me of a remorseful truth—I survived cancer, but my younger sister, Janet, did not.

But what most disturbed me about taking on the identity of a cancer survivor was something else entirely. I feared being subjected to the stigma placed on me by others in my social and professional network. I especially did not want my academic colleagues to think of me as someone who was on her way out, who wouldn't be in the academic profession for long. Shortly after my sister died, I remember running into a colleague at another university who talked about a mutual friend of ours in her department. This friend had recently developed breast cancer and decided to undergo a double mastectomy. What I remember vividly was the horror on my colleague's face as she told me the story—she thought our mutual friend was going to die. I did not want to deal with the stigma that disclosing my diagnosis might entail. I especially did not want to be written off by my colleagues and others in my field (Goffman 1963). Instead, I engaged in what sociologist Erving Goffman terms "passing"—maintaining the illusion of normalcy to others in my life and acting as if everything was normal (79).

Because my cancer was treatable and in its early stages, I was able, for the most part, to incorporate my cancer treatment into my everyday routine and in this way, I was able to hide my cancer diagnosis from others. Sociologist Kathy Charmaz's (1991; 1995) research regarding the process by which individuals adapt to living with chronic illness, provided me with important insights into my own cancer illness and subsequent adaptation. Charmaz notes that the extent to which a chronic illness impacts one's sense of identity depends on its severity and duration. An individual's adaptation to chronic illness is therefore variable and changing and can range from ignoring or minimizing illness, to struggling against it and, at the advanced stages of severity, reconciling oneself to it and embracing it. The further along the severity of illness continuum, the more one's sense of identity becomes more and more defined by one's illness state (Charmaz 1995). Reflecting on my own response to my cancer diagnosis, I was, unlike my younger sister, able to minimize and preserve a sense of self; a wholeness between my body and the persona I projected to others and thereby keeping my sense of self (mind and body) intact. I could contain and I thought, neutralize my own cancer diagnosis. The women in my study who have tested positive for the BRCA mutation and are in that liminal space where they feel the gap between diagnosis and illness is shrinking, and by seeking surgery they also see this choice as also "containing" their illness. They in fact, as we have observed, come to believe they have destroyed any threat of cancer before it strikes them. They do not want to wait for cancer to come.

As I began the interviews for this project, I again faced the dilemma of the extent to which I should disclose my own cancer and genetic testing experience to the women I interviewed, especially to those who asked me directly why I was interested in doing this type of research. At first, I told them about my younger sister's death from stage IV breast cancer and that this study provided me with a way to honor her memory, as well as to utilize my research skills on behalf of BRCA-positive mutation women. When I did talk briefly about my own experience, I remember feeling very uncomfortable sharing this information with my respondents. However, as I continued to interview women and deeply listened to their stories, I began to relate more and more of my own lived experiences. I told them about being tested for the BRCA mutation, and sharing my experiences allowed me to connect with them and with what they were going through.

As the interviews proceeded, I began to reexperience the trauma of my younger sister's death. Especially when some women I interviewed began to tell their own stories of having lost sisters to breast cancer, it became harder for me to do the next interview. I used various techniques to continue listening to their very gripping emotional stories. I listened through a headset while lying down on the floor so as to have my hands free in order to feel more relaxed and less tense. I did yoga poses—anything to get through the sometimes very painful accounts of their lives.

Humor was another tool that helped me cope with such emotionally and personally trying topics. Humor allowed both me and my respondent to step back from a woman's story and actually see some of the ridiculousness of a given situation. I can remember one of these moments vividly, when a woman commented on her new boyfriend's reaction to the news that, as she put it, "My boobs were fake." She was able to see the humor in that particular revelation, and wielded it to cut through her fear that he might decide to turn away from her.

About eleven interviews into my project, it was almost as if I hit a brick wall. I felt I could not do one more interview. Upon reflecting on my own interview experience during those eleven interviews, I thought I was practicing reflexivity about the interview process. I'd write memos about themes I considered important in a particular interview; I'd make extensive notes on new ideas coming out of the interviews, ideas I could follow up in subsequent interviews; and I reflected on whose voices were missing from my sample and considered how to obtain a more diverse group of women by age, marital status, race, ethnicity, and so on. What I didn't see, however, was the emotional toll these interviews were taking on me. I powerfully remember the comments of one woman I interviewed early on in the study. "Well, Sharlene," she asked, "how are you holding up doing the interviews with folks like me?" And I was surprised by her question then. At that point in my project, I really felt my own cancer and BRCA-testing experiences were only advantages because they allowed me to connect to these women. I was also careful not to interpret their experiences as if they were the same as mine.

Thinking back to those first eleven interviews, I realize, now, that I didn't check in on my own emotional barometer enough, partly because, as I noted earlier, I really didn't want to identify with my own cancer diagnosis and the cancer history that had affected my family. I became good at hiding these difficult feelings from myself. Once I stopped interviewing, I felt that this would be the end of the project, since it was just too difficult for me to do this type of emotionally charged work given my history. So, for about five months, I gave myself an emotional break from the project, hoping I could work through my feelings about cancer and my emotional response to what had happened to my family and me. I somehow came to terms with what I realized was my new normal. Part of that new normal was acknowledging my past and allowing myself to feel these emotions and the fear that my respondents had shared, especially the fear of waiting for cancer to return.

If someone were to ask me exactly how I restarted my project, I could not say, exactly. I'm still not sure what allowed me to find the emotional energy to continue. What I can say is that, by confronting my own emotional trauma, I was able to place what happened to me in perspective. This process took about five months. After that time, I felt I had somehow turned an emotional corner that allowed me to restart my project. I also overcame my concerns about disclosing my story to those respondents who wanted to know more about my specific interest in the project, and I began to share part of my own cancer journey and genetic-testing experience when it seemed appropriate for the interview. I especially shared my story when my respondent might have felt as if she had revealed too much of her personal story to me. It was as if I needed to balance the disclosing of information between interviewer and interviewee. Making this personal connection by sharing my story opened up a wider space of trust, so interviewees were willing to disclose more. When I look back at the interviews, I see my own self-disclosure was variable. I think after I made the decision to tell more of my own story, I did so as a way of challenging my own emotional boundaries. I gradually shared less because I worried that disclosing so much of my story might take a bit away from my respondent's story. Once I wasn't struggling with this issue on a personal level, I could follow the lead of my respondents—what did they want to know about my life? If someone asked me a direct question about my own history, I answered it. What I said about my cancer and BRCA history depended on my respondents' reactions and questions.

At times, just revealing some personal information, such as my sister dying of breast cancer, would be enough to explain my motivation for the study. Disclosing any more details about my situation, I thought, might take away from my role of listening to a woman's story. However, by telling a bit of my own story, I also brought a new type of energy and authenticity to the project. And I feel that accepting my new normal and incorporating my story into the interviews allowed me to engage more fully with the interview process as a whole.

The Pink Underside: A Parting Thought

I reflected on why it was that I never felt a part of the "pink ribbon culture" and instead continue to steer clear of this form of biosociality. Part of my reluctance to join it lay beyond feeling stigmatized or afraid of others' the negative reactions to my diagnosis. Instead, I experienced a feeling of not fitting into what I saw was the unitary upbeat portrayal of illness on cancer support group websites: the "pink-ribbon breast cancer cult" Ehrenreich described during her own experiences as a cancer survivor. One woman articulated this idea of the "gift" of cancer when she explained to Ehrenrich, "breast cancer has given me a new life. Breast cancer was something I needed to experience to open my eyes to the joy of living." (Ehrenreich 2010). Ehrenreich's response to her cancer was one of anger toward the medical and pharmaceutical industry that had recommended she take hormone replacement therapy, a fact she felt played a significant role in her own cancer diagnosis. Yet these support groups did not greet her anger with support; rather, they marginalized her cancer experience. She went on to note that the "cheerfulness of breast cancer culture goes beyond mere absence of anger to what looks, all too often, like a positive embrace of the disease" (Ehrenreich 2010).

What the women in my study taught me is that there are a multitude of reactions and adjustments to being a BRCA-positive mutation carrier and/ or cancer survivor. They consist a range of ongoing physical and emotional upheavals, as well as changes to one's relational networks. For some women, their belief that their own "cancer is a gift," or "BRCA is a gift," is one reaction of many in the face of illness, recovery, and the fear of dying. Ehrenreich's concern lies in the inability of the pink ribbon culture to accept and validate the wide range of women's reactions and concerns on multiple levels, including the role that corporate environmental polluters play in causing the rising rates of breast and ovarian cancer. Some of these corporations, may in fact, provide financial support to these same support groups and foundations (Ehrenreich 2010).

Women's lived experiences are complex and embodied. One's experience is relational and embedded in the web of social relations of everyday life. But when one hegemonic ideal of what a breast and/or ovarian cancer or BRCA experience should be—upbeat, positive, optimistic—dominates the medical and professional discourse and the media advertising, this pushes aside those whose experiences are just as valid, and need to be recognized, addressed and respected.

I attempt to look at the multiple levels of experiential reality, and this problem posed by the pink ribbon culture ignores such multiple realities.

Sharing Women's Stories

In writing this book, I employed a feminist standpoint approach to develop the most in-depth portrayal of women's stories. With a team of undergraduate research assistants, I took a grounded approach at all levels, so as to be open to new and conflicting ideas. As a team, my assistants and I challenged each other to describe, and to analyze and interpret women's stories using a grounded theory approach. More than one research assistant read each interview. They analyzed some themes by writing memos that compared and contrasted women's lived experiences. I gathered each of these memos together and wrote a comprehensive memo for each interview that drew on some of these observations. I focused on analyzing women's stories without using extensive computer-assisted software analysis programs in order to keep these stories whole, and to eliminate layers of analysis that might come between the specific multianalytical methods and women's lived experiences.

Completing a book like this would not have been possible without the amazing contributions of each woman I interviewed, as well as cross-checking demographics with the survey data. My research design allowed me to first use the in-depth interviews to explore women's experiences and iteratively develop themes, trends, as well as to develop new questions to ask in later interviews. I was also able to create an online survey based on the in-depth interviews that will form the basis of a larger online survey of both men and women's BRCA-positive mutation experiences pre- and post-testing. The data derived from the surveys also allowed me to do member-checking with regard to demographic information on women's family cancer history, as well as to cross-check some of the themes identified in the grounded theory analysis of the interviews. A literature review on the topics of BRCA testing and the genetic testing industry as a whole rounded out the project. My engagement with the research literature revealed the wider social, medical, commercial, and cultural contexts of women's experiences, which many women had alluded to, as we saw in chapters 1 and 7. By weaving women's narratives with academic research, I sought to give credence to every woman who spoke with me while also looking at the wider cultural influences that affected their experiences and decisions.

I hope this book is informative to women going through the BRCA experience, to professionals in the field of genetic research, and to the population in general, and I hope that the women who spoke with me are seen in this book to be speaking for themselves. My experience and biases inevitably have influenced the words and stories I chose to relate, but, to the greatest extent possible, and by working on each chapter with a research team that helped me tell these women's stories, I have aimed to portray accurately and sensitively the experiences of BRCA-positive mutation women.

Bibliography

American Civil Liberties Union (ACLU). 2013. "ACLU Challenges Patents on Breast Cancer Genes: BRCA." http://www.aclu.org/free-speech-womens-rights/aclu-challenges-patents-breast-cancer-genes-0.

Andersen, M. R., D. J. Bowen, J. Morea, K. D. Stein, and F. Baker. 2009. "Involvement in Decision-Making and Breast Cancer Survivor Quality of Life." *Health Psychology* 28(1): 29–37.

Anzaldu'a, G. 1987. *Borderlands/la frontera: The New Mestiza.* San Francisco: Spinsters/ Aumt Lute.

Arman, M., and A. Rehnsfeldt. 2003. "The Hidden Suffering Among Breast Cancer Patients: A Qualitative Metasynthesis." *Qualitative Health Research* 13(4): 510–27.

Armstrong, D. 1995. "The Rise of Surveillance Medicine." *Sociology of Health & Illness.* (17): 393–404.

Aronowitz, Robert A. 2009. "The Converged Experience of Risk and Disease." *Milbank Quarterly.* 87(2): 417–42.

Aronowitz, Robert A. 2010. "Decision Making and Fear in the Midst of Life." *Lancet* 375(9724): 1430–31.

Atkinson, P. A. 1997. *The Clinical Experience: The Construction and Reconstruction of Medical Reality.* 2nd edition. Aldershot: Ashgate.

Atkinson, P. H., H. Greenslade, and P. Glasner, eds. 2007. *New Genetics, New Identities.* New York: Routledge.

Atkinson, P. H., and P. Glasner. 2007. "Introduction: New Genetic Identities?" In *New Genetics, New Identities,* edited by P. H. Atkinson, H. Greenslade, and P. Glasner, 1–10. New York: Routledge.

Atkinson, P. H., P. Glasner, and M. Lock. 2009. *The Handbook of Genetics & Society: Mapping the New Genomic Era.* New York: Routledge.

Babb, Sheri A., Elizabeth M. Swisher, Hope N. Heller, Alison J. Whelan, David G. Mutch, Thomas J. Herzog, and Janet S. Rader. 2002. "Qualitative Evaluation of Medical Information Processing Needs of 60 Women Choosing Ovarian Cancer Surveillance or Prophylactic Oophorectomy." *Journal of Genetic Counseling* 11(2): 81–96.

Beck, U. 1992. *Risk Society: Toward a New Modernity.* Thousand Oaks, CA: Sage.

Begg, Colin B., Robert W. Haile, Åke Borg, Kathleen E. Malone, Patrick Concannon,

Duncan C. Thomas, Bryan Langholz, Leslie Bernstein, Jørgen H. Olsen, Charles F. Lynch, Hoda Anton-Culver, Marinela Capanu, Xiaolin Liang, Amanda J. Hummer, Cami Sima, and Jonine L. Bernstein. 2008. "Variation of Breast Cancer Risk among *BRCA1/2* Carriers." *Journal of American Medical Association* 299(2): 194–201.

Bermejo-Perez, M. J., S. Márquez-Calderón, and A. Llanos-Méndez. 2007. "Effectiveness of Preventive Interventions in BRCA1/2 Gene Mutation Carriers: A Systematic Review." *International Journal of Cancer* 121(2): 225–31.

Bluman, Leslie G., Barbara Rimer, Katherine R. Sterba, Julia Lancaster, Shelley Clark, Nancy Borstelmann, J. Dirk Iglehard, and Eric P. Winer. 2003. "Attitudes, Knowledge, Risk Perceptions and Decision-Making among Women with Breast and/or Ovarian Cancer Considering Testing for BRCA1 and BRCA2 and their Spouses." *Psycho-Oncology* 12: 410–27.

Bowen, Deborah J., Kathryn M. Battuello, and Monique Raats. 2005. "Marketing Genetic Tests: Empowerment or Snake Oil?" *Health Education & Behavior* 32(5): 676–85.

Brierly, K. L., D. Campfield, W. Ducaine, L. Dohany, T. Donenberg, K. Shannon, R. C. Schwartz, and E. T. Matloff. 2010. "Errors in Delivery of Cancer Genetic Services: Implications for Practice." *Connecticut Medicine* 74(7): 413–23.

Brower, Vicki. 2010. "FDA to Regulate Direct-to-Consumer Genetic Tests." *Journal of the National Cancer Institute* 102(21): 1610–17.

Brown, S. M., et al. 2011. "Health Literacy, Numeracy, and Interpretation of Graphical Breast Cancer Risk Estimates." *Patient Education and Counseling* 83(1): 92–98.

Browner, Carole H., and H. Mabel Preloran. 2010. *Neurogenetic Diagnoses: The Power of Hope and the Limits of Today's Medicine.* New York: Routledge.

Bryant, T., and C. Charmaz. 2007. *Handbook of Grounded Theory.* Thousand Oaks, CA: Sage.

Burke, C. S., and C. J. Castaneda. 2007. "The Public and Private History of Eugenics: An Introduction." *Public Historian* 29(3): 5–17.

Burke, W. 2004. "Genetic Testing in Primary Care." *Annual Review of Genomics and Human Genetics* 5: 1–14.

Butler, Judith. 1990. *Gender Trouble: Feminism and the Subversion of Identity.* New York: Routledge.

"Cancer Previvors: Overview." FORCE: Facing Our Risk of Cancer Empowered. http://www.facingourrisk.org/info_research/previvors-survivors/cancer-previvors/index.php. Accessed March 1, 2012.

Cancer Risk Assessment. "About Us." www.cancerriskassessment.com. Accessed June 12, 2010.

Carroll, P., K. Dew, and P. Howden-Chapman. 2011. "The Heart of the Matter: Using Poetry as a Method of Ethnographic Inquiry to Represent and Present Experiences of the Informally Housed in Aotearoa/New Zealand." *Qualitative Inquiry* 17(7): 623–30.

Cathy. "Why Take a Breast Cancer/Ovarian Cancer Risk Assessment Test?" Myriad Genetics. http://www.bracnow.com/considering-testing/why-take-a-breast-ovarian-cancer-risk-test.php.

Chalmers, K., and K. Thomson. 1996. "Coming to Terms with the Risk of Breast Cancer: Perceptions of Women with Primary Relatives with Breast Cancer." *Qualitative Health Research* 6: 256–82.

Charmaz, K. 1991. *Good Days, Bad Days: The Self in Chronic Illness and Time.* New Brunswick, NJ: Rutgers University Press.

Charmaz, K. 1995. "The Body, Identity, and Self: Adapting to Impairment." *Sociological Quarterly* 36(4): 657–80.

Charmaz, K. 2006. *Constructing Grounded Theory: A Practical Guide Through Qualitative Analysis.* Thousand Oaks, CA: Sage.

Claes, Erna, Gerry Evers-Kiebooms, Andrea Boogaerts, Marleen Decruyenaere, Lieve Denayer, and Eric Legius. 2003. "Communication with Close and Distant Relatives in the context of Genetic Testing for Hereditary Breast and Ovarian Cancer in Cancer Patients." *American Journal of Medical Genetic* 116A(1): 11–19.

Clarke, Adele E., Jennifer Ruth Fosket, Laura Mamo, Janet K. Shim, and Jennifer R. Fishman, eds. 2010. *Biomedicalization: Technoscience, Health and Illness in the U.S.* Durham, NC: Duke University Press.

Clarke, Adele E., Laura Mamo, Janet K. Shim, Jennifer Ruth Fosket, and Jennifer R. Fishman. 2003. "Biomedicalization: Technoscientific Transformations of Health, Illness, and U.S. Biomedicine." *American Sociological Review* 68(2): 161–94.

Collins, P. H. 1990. *Black Feminist Thought: Knowledge, Consciousness, and the Politics of Empowerment.* New York: Routledge.

Companies and Markets. "Overview: The genetic testing market is expected to grow at a CAGR of 7.2%." http://www.companiesandmarkets.com/Market/Healthcare-and-Medical/Market-Research/Genetic-Testing-Reagents-Global-Pipeline-Analysis-Competitive-Landscape-and-Market-Forecasts-to-2017/RPT937761.

Condit, Celeste M. 2010. "Public Attitudes and Beliefs about Genetics." *Annual Review of Genomics and Human Genetics* 11: 339–59.

Conrad, P., and Gabe, J., eds. 1999. *Sociological Perspectives on the New Genetics.* Oxford: Blackwell.

d'Agincourt-Canning, L. 2005. "The Effect of Experiential Knowledge on Construction of Risk Perception in Hereditary Breast/Ovarian Cancer." *Journal of Genetic Counseling* 14(1): 55–69.

d'Agincourt-Canning, L. 2006. "A Gift or a Yoke? Women's and Men's Responses to Genetic Risk Information from BRCA1 and BRCA2 Testing." *Clinical Genetics* 70: 462–72.

d'Agincourt-Canning, L., and P. Baird. 2006. "Genetic Testing for Hereditary Cancers: The Impact of Gender on Interest, Uptake and Ethical Considerations." *Critical Reviews in Oncology/Hematology* 58(2): 114–23.

Daly, Mary B. 2009. "The Impact of Social Roles on the Experience of Men in BRCA1/2 Families: Implications for Counseling." *Journal of Genetic Counseling* 18(1): 42–48.

Daly, Mary B., Andrea Barsevick, Suzanne M. Miller, Robert Buckman, Josephine Costalas, Susan Montgomery, and Ruth Bingler. 2001. "Communicating Genetic Test Results to the Family: A Six-Step, Skills-Building Strategy." *Family and Community Health* 24(3): 13–26.

Darwin, Charles. 2003 (1859). *The Origin of the Species: 150th Anniversary Edition.* New York: Signet Classics.

David Jay Photography. "The Scar Project: Breast Cancer is Not a Pink Ribbon." *The Scar Project.* http://www.thescarproject.org/.

De Leeuw, J. R. J., M. J. van Vliet, and M. G. Ausems. 2008. "Predictors of Choosing Life-Long Screening or Prophylactic Surgery in Women at High and Moderate Risk for Breast and Ovarian Cancer." *Familial Cancer* 7: 347–59.

de Vries-Kragt, K. 1998. "The Dilemmas of a Carrier of BRCA1 Gene Mutations." *Patient Education and Counseling* 35: 75–80.

Dhar, S. U., H. P. Cooper, T. Wang, B. Parks, S. A. Staggs, S. Hilsenbeck, and E. E. Plon. 2011. "Significant Differences among Physician Specialties in Management Recommendations of BRCA1 Mutation Carriers." *Breast Cancer Research and Treatment* 129(1): 221–27.

Douglas, Heather A., Rebekah J. Hamilton, and Robin E. Grubs. 2009. "The Effect of BRCA Gene Testing on Family Relationships: A Thematic Analysis of Qualitative Interviews." *Journal of Genetic Counseling* 18: 418–35.

Ehrenreich, B. 2010. *Bright-Sided: How Positive Thinking is Undermining America.* New York: Metropolitan Books/Henry Holt.

Erblich, Joel, Dana H. Bovbjerg, and Heiddis B. Valdismarsdottir. 2000. "Looking Forward and Back: Distress among Women at Familial Risk for Breast Cancer." *Annals of Behavior Medicine* 22(1): 53–62.

Finkler, K., C. Skrzynia, and J. P. Evans. 2003. "The New Genetics and its Consequences for Family, Kinship, Medicine and Medical Genetics." *Social Science and Medicine* 57(3): 403–12.

Forde, O. H. 1998. "Is Imposing Risk Awareness Cultural Imperialism?" *Social Science & Medicine* 47(9): 1155–59.

Forrest, K., S. A. Simpson, B. J. Wilson, E. R. van Teijlingen, L. McKee, N. Haites, and E. Matthews. 2003. "To Tell or Not to Tell: Barriers and Facilitators in Family Communication about Genetic Risk." *Clinical Genetics* 64: 317–26.

Fortuny, Daniel, Judith Balmaña, Begoña Graña, Asunción Torres, Teresa Ramón y Cajal, Esther Darder, and Neus Gadea. 2009. "Opinion about Reproductive Decision Making among Individuals Undergoing BRCA1/2 Genetic Testing in a Multicentre Spanish Cohort." *Human Reproduction* 24(4): 1000–1006.

Foucault, Michel. 1972. *The Archaeology of Knowledge.* Translated by A. M. Sheridan Smith. London: Tavistock.

Franklin, S., and C. Roberts. 2006. *Born and Made: An Ethnography of Preimplantation Genetic Diagnosis.* Princeton, NJ: Princeton University Press.

Gay, Alicia. "Today We Take Back Our Genes." American Civil Liberties Union (ACLU). http://www.aclu.org/blog/womens-rights-free-speech/today-we-take-back-our-genes.

Genetic Information Nondiscrimination Act (GINA) of 2008. National Human Genome Research Institute, National Institutes of Health. http://www.genome.gov/24519851.

Geransar, Rose, and Edna Einsiedel. 2008. "Evaluating Online Direct-to-Consumer Marketing of Genetic Tests: Informed Choices or Buyers Beware?" *Genetic Testing* 12(1): 13–23.

Gibbon, S. 2008. "Charity, Breast Cancer Activism and the Iconic Figure of the BRCA Carrier." In *Biosocialities, Genetics and the Social Sciences: Making Biologies and Identities* edited by S. Gibbon and C. Novas, 19–37. New York: Routledge.

Gibbon, S. and C. Novas, eds. 2008. *Biosocialities, Genetics and the Social Sciences: Making Biologies and Identities*. New York: Routledge.

Giddens, A. 1991. *Modernity and Self-Identity: Self and Society in the Late Modern Age*. Cambridge: Polity Press.

Glanz, K., B. K. Rimer, and F. M. Lewis. 2002. *Health Behavior and Health Education*. 3rd edition. New York: Jossey-Bass.

Glaser, Barney G., and Anselm L. Strauss. 1967. *The Discovery of Grounded Theory: Strategies for Qualitative Research*. Chicago: Aldine.

Goffman, E. 1963. *Stigma: Notes on the Management of Spoiled Identity*. New York: Prentice Hall.

Gold, Richard E., and Julia Carbone. 2010. "Myriad Genetics: In the Eye of the Policy Storm." *Genetics in Medicine* 12(4): S39–S70.

Gollust, Sarah E., Sara Chandros Hull, and Benjamin S. Wilfond. 2002. "Limitations of Direct-to-Consumer Advertising for Clinical Genetic Testing." *Journal of the American Medical Association* 288(14): 1762–67.

Hall, Allyson G., Amal J. Khoury, Ellen D. Lopez, Nedra Lisovicz, Amanda Avis-Williams, and Amal Mitra. 2008. "Breast Cancer Fatalism: The Role of Women's Perceptions of the Health Care System." *Journal of Health Care for the Poor and Underserved* 19: 1321–35.

Hall, Michael J., Julia E. Reid, Lynn A. Burbidge, Dmitry Pruss, Amie M. Deffenbaugh, Cynthia Frye, Richard J. Wenstrup, Brian E. Ward, Thomas A. Scholl, and Walter W. Noll. 2009. "BRCA1 and BRCA2 Mutations in Women of Different Ethnicities Undergoing Testing for Hereditary Breast-Ovarian Cancer." *Cancer* 15(10): 2222–33.

Hallowell, Nina. 1999. "Doing the Right Thing: Genetic Risk and Responsibility." *Sociology of Health & Illness* 21(5): 597–621.

Hallowell, Nina, A. Arden-Jones, R. Eeles, C. Foster, A. Lucassen, C. Moynihan, and M. Watson. 2005. "Men's Decision-Making about Predictive BRCA1/2 Testing: The Role of Family." *Journal of Genetic Counseling* 14(3): 207–17.

Hallowell, Nina, C. Foster, R. Eeles, A. Arden-Jones, V. Murday, and M. Watson. 2003. "Balancing Autonomy and Responsibility: The Ethics of Generating and Disclosing Genetic Information." *Journal of Medical Ethics* 29: 74–83.

Hallowell, Nina, I. Jacobs, M. Richards, J. Mackay, and M. Gore. 2001. "Surveillance or Surgery? A Description of the Factors that Influence High Risk Premenopausal Women's Decisions about Prophylactic Oophorectomy." *Journal of Medical Genetics* 38(10): 683–91.

Hallowell, Nina, and J. Lawton. 2002. "Negotiating Present and Future Selves: Managing the Risk of Hereditary Ovarian Cancer by Prophylactic Surgery." *Health: An Interdisciplinary Journal for the Social Study of Health, Illness and Medicine* 6(4): 423–43.

Hamilton, Rebekah, Janet K. Williams, Barbara J. Bowers, and Kathleen Calzone. 2009. "Life Trajectories, Genetic Testing, and Risk Reduction Decisions in 18–39 Year Old Women at Risk for Hereditary Breast and Ovarian Cancer." *Journal of Genetic Counseling* 18: 147–59.

Haraway, Donna. 1988. "Situated Knowledges: The Science Question in Feminism and the Privilege of Partial Perspective." *Feminist Studies* 14(3): 575–99.

Harding, Sandra. 1987. *Feminism and Methodology: Social Science Issues*. Bloomington: Indiana University Press.

"HBOC Basics." 2013. BRACAnalysis. http://www.bracnow.com/considering-testing/hboc-basics.php.

Hedgecoe, Adam. 2008. "The Personal Genome: Hopes, Facts, and Fears." European Bioinformatics Institute. http://www.ebi.ac.uk/Information/events/personalgenome/#abs3.

Herrnstein, Richard J., and Charles Murray. 1996. *Bell Curve: Intelligence and Class Structure in American Life.* New York: Free Press.

Heshka, J. T., C. Palleschi, H. Howley, B. Wilson, and P. S. Wells. 2008. "A Systematic Review of Perceived Risks, Psychological and Behavioral Impacts of Genetic Testing." *Genetics in Medicine* 10(1): 19–32.

Hesse-Biber, Sharlene. 2007. "Feminist Research: Exploring the Interconnections of Epistemology, Methodology and Methods." In *Feminist Research: Theory and Praxis,* edited by Sharlene Hesse-Biber, 1–28. Thousand Oaks, CA: Sage.

Hesse-Biber, Sharlene, and D. Piatelli. 2012. "The Feminist Practice of Holistic Reflexivity." In *The Handbook of Feminist Research: Theory and Praxis,* 2nd ed., edited by Sharlene Hesse-Biber, 493–514. Thousand Oaks, CA: Sage.

Holtzman, Neil A., and Michael S. Watson. 1997. "Promoting Safe and Effective Genetic Testing in the United States: Final Report of the Task Force on Genetic Testing." National Human Genome Research Institute. http://www.genome.gov/10001733.

Hogarth, Stuart, Gail Javitt, and David Melzer. 2008. "The CurrentL for Direct-to-Consumer Genetic Testing: Legal, Ethnical, and Policy Issues." *Annual Review of Genomics and Human Genetics* 9: 161–82.

hooks, bell. 1984. *Feminist Theory: From Margin to Center.* Boston: South End Press.

Hopwood, P., A. Lee, A. Shenton, A. Baildam, A. Brain, F. Lalloo, G. Evans, and A. Howell, A. 2000. "Clinical Follow-Up after Bilateral Risk Reducing ('Prophylactic') Mastectomy: Mental Health and Body Image Outcomes." *Psycho-Oncology* 9(6): 462–72.

Hoskins, Lindsey M., Kevin Roy, June A. Peters, Jennifer T. Loud, and Mark H. Greene. 2008. "Disclosure of Positive BRCA1/2-Mutation Status in Young Couples: The Journey from Uncertainty to Bonding through Partner Support." *Families, Systems, & Health* 26(3): 296–316.

Howard, A. Fuchsia, J. L. Bottorff, L. G. Balneaves, and C. Kim-Sing. 2010. "Women's Constructions of the 'Right Time' to Consider Decisions about Risk-Reducing Mastectomy and Risk-Reducing Oophorectomy." *BMC Women's Health* 10(24): 1–12.

Howard, A. Fuchsia, Lynda G. Balneaves, and Joan L. Bottorff. 2009. "Women's Decision Making about Risk-Reducing Strategies in the Context of Hereditary Breast and Ovarian Cancer: A Systematic Review." *Journal of Genetic Counseling* 18: 578–97.

Huff, Charlotte. "The Genes that Bind." *Cure.* http://www.curetoday.com/index.cfm/fuseaction/article.show/id/2/article_id/1483.

Hughes, L., and C. Phelps. 2010. "'The Bigger the Network the Bigger the Bowl of Cherries . . .' : Exploring the Acceptability of, and Preferences for, an Ongoing Support Network for Known BRCA 1 and BRCA 2 Mutation Carriers." *Journal of Genetic Counseling* 19(5): 487–96.

Hull, Sara, and Kiran Prasad. 2001. "Reading Between the Lines: Direct-to-Consumer Advertising of Genetic Testing in the USA." *Reproductive Health Matters* 9(18): 44–48.

Isaacs, C., B. N. Peshkin, M. Schwartz, T. A. DeMarco, D. Main, and C. Lerman. 2002. "Breast and Ovarian Cancer Screening Practices in Healthy Women with a Strong Family History of Breast or Ovarian Cancer." *Breast Cancer Research and Treatment* 71: 103–12.

Julian-Reynier, Claire, François Eisinger, François Chabal, Christine Lasset, Catherine Noguès, Dominique Stoppa-Lyonnet, Philippe Vennin, and Hagay Sobol. 2000. "Disclosure to the Family of Breast/Ovarian Cancer Genetic Test Results: Patient's Willingness and Associated factors." *American Journal of Medical Genetics* 94: 13–18.

Kelly, D. 2009. "Changed Men: The Embodied Impact of Prostate Cancer." *Qualitative Health Research* 19(2): 151–63.

Kenen, R. H. 1994. "The Human Genome Project: Creator of the Potentially Sick, Potentially Vulnerable and Potentially Stigimatised?" In *Life and Death Under High Technology Medicine,* edited by Ian Robinson, 49–64. Manchester: Manchester University Press.

Kenen R. H., A. Arden-Hones, and R. Eeles. 2003. "Family Stories and the Use of Heuristics: Women from Suspected Hereditary Breast and Ovarian Cancer (HBOC) Families." *Sociology of Health & Illness* 25(7): 838–65.

Kenen, R. H., P. J. Shapiro, L. Hantsoo, S. Fridman, and J. C. Coyne. 2007. "Women with *BRCA1* or *BRCA2* Mutations Renegotiating a Post-Prophylactic Mastectomy Identity: Self-Image and Self-Disclosure." *Journal of Genetic Counseling* 16: 789–98.

Klitzman, Robert. 2010. "Views of Discrimination among Individuals Confronting Genetic Disease." *Journal of Genetic Counseling* 19: 68–83.

Klitzman, Robert L., and Meghan M. Sweeney. 2011. "'In Sickness and in Health'? Disclosures of Genetic Risks in Dating." *Journal of Genetic Counseling* 20(1): 98–112.

Koehly, L. M., J. A. Peters, N. Kuhn, L. Hoskins, A. Letocha, R. Kenen, J. Loud, and M. H. Greene. 2008. "Sisters in Hereditary Breast and Ovarian Cancer Families: Communal Coping, Social Integration, and Psychological Well-Being." *Psycho-Oncology* 17: 812–21.

Kurian, Allison W., Bronislava M. Sigal, and Sylvia K. Plevritis. 2010. "Survival Analysis of Cancer Risk Reduction Strategies for *BRCA1/2* Mutation Carriers." *Journal of Clinical Oncology* 28(2) 222–31.

Lagos, Veronica I., Matrin A. Perez, Charité N Ricker, Kathleen R. Blazer, Nydia M. Santiago, Nancy Feldman, Lori Viveros, and Jeffrey N. Weitzel. 2008. "Social-Cognitive Aspects of Underserved Latinas Preparing to Undergo Genetic Cancer Risk Assessment for Hereditary Breast and Ovarian Cancer." *Psycho-Oncology* 17: 774–82.

Leachman, Stacy A., Daniel G. MacArthur, Misha Angrist, Stacy W. Gray, Angela R. Bradbury, and Daniel B. Vorhaus. 2011. "Direct-to-Consumer Genetic Testing: Personalized Medicine in Evolution." *American Society of Clinical Oncology 2011 Educational Book.* 34–40.

Lee, Sandra Soo-Jin. 2009. "Social networking in the age of personal genomics." *Saint Louis University Journal of Health Law & Policy* 3(1): 41–60.

Lee, Simon J. Craddock. 2010. "Uncertain Futures: Individual Risk and Social Context in Decision-Making in Cancer Screening." *Health, Risk & Society* 12(2): 101–17.

Lerman, Caryn, C. Hughes, R. T. Croyle, D. Main, C. Durham, C. Snyder, A. Bonney, J. F. Lynch, S. A. Narod, and H. T. Lynch. 2000. "Prophylactic Surgery Decisions and Surveillance Practices One Year Following BRCA1/2 Testing." *Preventive Medicine* 32(1): 75–80.

Lerman, Caryn, Janet Seay, Andrew Balshem, and Janet Audrain. 1995. "Interest in Genetic Testing among First-Degree Relatives of Breast Cancer Patients." *American Journal of Medical Genetics* 57: 385–92.

Levy-Lahad, E., and E. Friedman. 2007. "Cancer Risks among BRCA1 and BRCA2 Mutation Carriers." *British Journal of Cancer* 96: 11–15.

Lewis, P. J. 2011. "Storytelling as Research/Research as Storytelling." *Qualitative Inquiry* 17(6): 505–10.

Lincoln, Y. S. 1995. "Emerging Criteria for Quality in Qualitative and Interpretive Research." *Qualitative Inquiry* 1(3): 275–89.

Lippman, Abby. 1991. "Prenatal Genetic Testing and Screening: Constructing Needs and Reinforcing Inequities." *American Journal of Law & Medicine* 17(1–2): 15–50.

Litton, J. K., S. N, Westin, K. Ready, C. C. Sun, S. K. Peterson, F. Meric-Bernstam, A. M. Gonzalez-Angulo, D. C. Bordurka, K. H. Lu, G. N. Kortobagyi, and B. K. Arun. 2009. "Perception of Screening and Risk Reduction Surgeries in Patients Tested for a BRCA Deleterious Mutation." *Cancer* 115(8): 1598–604.

Liu, Yuping, and Yvette E. Pearson. 2008. "Direct-to-Consumer Marketing of Predictive Medical Genetic Tests: Assessment of Current Practices and Policy Recommendations." *American Marketing Association* 27(2): 131–48.

Lloyd, S. M., M. Watson, G. Oaker, N. Sacks, U. Querci Della Rovere, and G. Gui. 2000. "Understanding the Experience of Prophylactic Bilateral Mastectomy: A Qualitative Study of Ten Women." *Psycho-Oncology* 9: 473–85.

Lowstuter, K. J., S. Sand, K. R. Blazer, D. J. MacDonald, K. C. Banks, C. A. Lee, B. U. Schwerin, M. Juarez, G. C. Uman, and J. N. Weitzel. 2008. "Influence of Genetic Discrimination Perceptions and Knowledge on Cancer Genetics Referral Practice among Clinicians." *Genetics in Medicine* 10(9): 691–98.

Lupton, D., ed. 1999. *Risk and Sociocultural Theory: New Directions and Perspectives.* Cambridge: Cambridge University Press.

Lydersen, Kari. 2010. "Date against Time." *Time Out Chicago.* http://timeoutchicago.com/sex-dating/74344/date-against-time.

MacKenzie, Amy, Linda Patrick-Miller, and Angela R. Bradbury. 2009. "Controversies in Communication of Genetic Risk for Hereditary Breast Cancer." *Breast Journal* 15(1): 25–32.

Mahon, S. M. 2011. "Impact of the Genetic Screening Revolution: Understanding and Meeting the Needs of Previvors with a Known Family Mutation in BRCA/BRCA2." *Evidence-Based Nursing* 14: 126–27.

Manderson, L., and S. Peake. 2005. "Boundary Breaches: The Body, Sex and Sexuality Post-Stoma Surgery." *Social Science and Medicine* 61(2): 405–15.

Mann, S. A., and L. R. Kelly. 1997. "Standing at the Crossroads of Modernist Thought: Collins, Smith, and the New Feminist Epistemologies." *Gender & Society* 11(4): 391–408.

Martin, P. 1995. "The American Gene Therapy Industry and the Social Shaping of a New Technology." *Genetic Engineer and Biotechnologist* 15: 155–67.

Matloff, Ellen, and Arthur Caplan. 2008. "Direct to Confusion: Lessons Learned from Marketing BRCA Testing." *American Journal of Bioethics* 8(6): 5–8.

Matrix Genomics. n.d. "Personal Genomics to Enhance your Life and Life Expectancy!" http://www.matrixgenomics.com/index.php.

McCabe, L. L., and E. R. B. McCabe. 2004. "Direct-to-Consumer Genetic Testing: Access and Marketing." *Genetics in Medicine* 6(1): 58–59.

McGivern, G., et al. 2004. "Family Communication about Positive BRCA1 and BRCA2 Genetic Test Results." *Genetics in Medicine* 6(6): 503–9.

Mellon, S., J. Janisse, R. Gold, M. Cichon, L. Berry-Bobovski, M. A. Tainsky, and M. S. Simon. 2009. "Predictors of Decision Making in Families at Risk for Inherited Breast/Ovarian Cancer." *Health Psychology* 28(1): 38–47.

Menon, U., J. Harper, A. Sharma, L. Fraser, M. Burnell, K. El Masry, C. Rodeck, and I. Jacobs. 2007. "Views of BRCA Gene Mutation Carriers on Preimplantation Genetic Diagnosis as a Reproductive Option for Hereditary Breast and Ovarian Cancer." *Human Reproductive* 22(6): 1573–77.

Metcalfe, K. A., and S. A. Narod. 2002. "Breast Cancer Risk Perception among Women Who Have Undergone Prophylactic Bilateral Mastectomy." *Journal of the National Cancer Institute* 94(20): 1564–69.

Moersky, J. 2012. *Risky Genes: Genetics, breast cancer and jewish identity*. New York: Routledge.

Mogilner, Avigyail, Marc Otten, John D. Cunningham, and Steven T. Brower. 1998. "Awareness and Attitudes Concerning BRCA Gene Testing." *Annals of Surgical Oncology* 5(7): 607–12.

Mohanty, C. 1988. "Under Western Eyes: Feminist Scholarship and Colonial Discourses." *Feminist Review* 30(1): 61–88.

Mor, Pnina, and Kathleen Oberle. 2008. "Issues Related to BRCA Gene Testing in Orthodox Jewish Women." *Nursing Ethics* 15(4): 512–22.

Myriad Genetics. 2013. "BRACAnalysis." www.bracnow.com.

Myriad Genetics. 2007. "Myriad Genetics: Annual Report 2007." http://www.myriad.com/downloads/Myriad-Annual-Report-2007.pdf.

Myriad Genetics. 2007. "Myriad Genetics Launches Awareness Advertising Campaign to Educate Women about Hereditary Risks of Breast and Ovarian Cancers." http://investor.myriad.com/releasedetail.cfm?ReleaseID=325769.

Myriad Genetics. 2011. "Myriad Genetics Reports Fiscal 2011 Third Quarter Results: Record Third Quarter Revenue of $102.4 Million and Operating Income of $41.8 Million." http://investor.myriad.com/releasedetail.cfm?releaseid=574140.

Myriad Genetics. 2012. "Myriad Genetics Reports Second Quarter Fiscal Year 2012 Results." http://investor.myriad.com/releasedetail.cfm?ReleaseID=644317.

Narayan, D., ed. 2005. *Measuring Empowerment: Cross-Disciplinary Perspectives*. Washington, D.C.: World Bank.

National Cancer Institute. 2009. "BRCA1 and BRCA2: Cancer Risk and Genetic Testing." http://www.cancer.gov/cancertopics/factsheet/Risk/BRCA.

National Cancer Institute. 2012. "Genetics of Breast and Ovarian Cancer (PDQ)." http://www.cancer.gov/cancertopics/pdq/genetics/breast-and-ovarian/HealthProfessional.

Nelson, Heidi D., Laurie Hoyt Huffman, Rongwie Fu, Emily L. Harris, Miranda Walker, and Christina Bougatsos. 2005. "Genetic Risk Assessment and BRCA Mutation Testing for Breast and Ovarian Cancer Susceptibility: Evidence Synthesis." Prepared for Agency for Healthcare Research and Quality, U.S. Department of Health and Human Services. http://www.ahrq.gov/downloads/pub/prevent/pdfser/brcagensyn.pdf.

Nelson, J. J., J. Gould, and S. Keller-Olaman, eds. 2009. *Cancer on the Margins: Method and Meaning in Participatory Research.* Toronto: University of Toronto Press.

North, Kari E., and Lisa J. Martin. 2008. "The Importance of Gene-Environmental Interaction: Implications for Social Scientists." *Sociological Methods & Research* 37(2): 164–200.

Novas, Carlos, and Nikolas Rose. 2000. "Genetic Risk and the Birth of the Somatic Individual." *Economy and Society* 29(4): 485–514.

O'Connor, Shelia. 2010. "Top News: Walgreens Postpones Carrying Genetic Test Kit." Examiner.com. http://www.examiner.com/sf-in-san-francisco/top-news-walgreens-postpones-carrying-genetic-test-kit-photos.

Oliffe, J. 2006. "Embodied Masculinity and Androgen Deprivation Therapy." *Sociology of Health & Illness* 2(4): 410–32.

Ormondroyd, E., L. Donnelly, C. Moynihan, C. Savona, E. Bancroft, D. G. Evans, R. A. Eeles, S. Lavery, and M. Watson. 2011. "Attitudes to Reproductive Genetic Testing in Women Who Had a Positive BRCA Test Before Having Children: A Qualitative Analysis." *European Journal of Human Genetics* 20(1): 1–7.

Ossorio, Pilar, and Troy Duster. 2005. "Race and Genetics: Controversies in Biomedical, Behavioral, and Forensic Sciences." *American Psychological Association* 60(1): 115–28.

Ozanne, E. M., et al. 2009. "Identification and Management of Women at High Risk for Hereditary Breast/Ovarian Cancer Syndrome." *Breast Journal* 15(2): 155–62.

Patenaude, A. F., M. Dorval, L. S. DiGianni, K. A. Schneider, A. Chittenden, and Judy E. Garber. 2006. "Sharing BRCA1/2 Test Results with First-Degree Relatives: Factors Predicting Who Women Tell." *Journal of Clinical Oncology* 24(4): 700–706.

Peshkin, Beth N., Tiffani A. DeMarco, and Kenneth P. Tercyak. 2010. "On the Development of a Decision Support Intervention for Mothers Undergoing *BRCA1/2* Cancer Genetic Testing Regarding Communicating Rest Results to their Children." *Familial Cancer* 9: 89–97.

Pilarski, Robert. 2009. "Risk Perception among Women at Risk for Hereditary Breast and Ovarian Cancer." *Journal of Genetic Counseling* 18: 303–12.

Pinto, Barbara. 2007. "Split Realities for Sisters with Breast Cancer Gene." *ABC World News*, October 8. http://a.abcnews.com/WN/OnCallPlus/story?id=3704741&page=1.

Pollack, Andrew. 2007. "A Genetic Test that Very Few Need, Marketed to the Masses." *New York Times*, September 11.

Pollack, Andrew. 2012. "Justices Send Back Gene Case." *New York Times*, March 26.

Portnoy, D. B., D. Roter, and L. H. Erby. 2010. "The Role of Numeracy on Client Knowledge in BRCA Genetic Counseling." *Patient Education and Counseling* 81(1): 131–36.

Potts, L. K., ed. 2000. *Ideologies of Breast Cancer: Feminist Perspectives.* New York: St. Martin's.

Pruthi, Sandhya, Bobbie S. Gostout, and Noralane M. Lindor. 2010. "Identification and Management of Women with BRCA Mutations or Hereditary Predisposition for Breast and Ovarian Cancer." *Mayo Clinic Proceedings* 85(12): 1111–20.

Quinn, G. P., et al. 2010. "BRCA Carriers' Thoughts on Risk Management in Relation to Preimplantation Genetic Diagnosis and Childbearing: When Too Many Choices Are Just as Difficult as None." *Fertility and Sterility* 94(6): 2473–75.

Rabinow, Paul. 1992. "Artificiality and Enlightenment: From Sociobiology to Biosociality." In *Anthropologies of Modernity: Foucault, Governmentality, and Life Politics,* edited by Jonathan Xavier Inda, 181–93. Oxford: Wiley-Blackwell.

Rodney, P., M. Burgess, G. McPherson, and H. Brown. 2004. "Our Theoretical Landscape: A Brief History of Health Care Ethics." In *Toward a Moral Horizon: Nursing Ethics for Leadership and Practice,* edited by J. Storch, P. Rodney and R. Starzomski, 56–97. Toronto: Pearson-Prentice Hall.

Rosenberg, Charles. 2009. "The Art of Medicine: Managed Fear." *Lancet* 373: 802–3.

Rothman, B. K. 1998. "Reproductive Technology and the Commodification of Life." *Women Health* 12(1–2): 95–100.

Sagi, M., N. Weinberg, A. Eilat, E. Aizenman, M. Werner, E. Girsh, Y. Siminovsky, D. Abeliovich, T. Peretz, A. Simon, and N. Laufer. 2009. "Preimplantation Genetic Diagnosis for BRCA1/2—A Novel Clinical Experience." *Prenatal Diagnosis* 29: 508–13.

Salant, T., P. S. Ganschow, O. I. Olopade, and D. S. Lauderdale. 2006. "'Why Take it if You Don't Have Anything?' Breast Cancer Risk Perceptions and Prevention Choices at a Public Hospital." *Journal of General Internal Medicine* 21(7): 779–85.

Shaffer, L. G., and I. B. den Veyver. 2012. "New Technologies for the Assessment of Chromosomes in Prenatal Diagnosis." *Prenatal Diagnosis* 32(4): 307–8.

Shuren, Jeffrey. 2010. "Direct-to-Consumer Genetic Testing and the Consequences to the Public. Statement before the Subcommittee on Oversight and Investigations Committee on Energy and Commerce, U.S. House of Representatives." FDA: U.S. Food and Drug Administration. http://www.fda.gov/NewsEvents/Testimony/ucm219925.htm.

Sivell, S., G. Elwyn, C. L. Gaff, A. J. Clarke, R. Iredale, C. Shaw, J. Dudon, H. Thornton, and A. Edwards. 2008. "How Risk is Perceived, Constructed and Interpreted by Clients in Clinical Genetics, and the Effects on Decision Making: Systematic Review." *Journal of Genetic Counseling* 17(1): 30–63.

Smith, Dorothy. 1987. *The Everyday World as Problematic: A Feminist Sociology.* Boston: Northeastern University Press.

Sorenson, J. R., and J. R. Botkin. 2003. "Introduction- Genetic Testing and the Family." *American Journal of Medical Genetics Part C: Seminars in Medical Genetics* 119C(1): 1–2.

Steinberg, Deborah Lynn. 1997. *Bodies in Glass: Genetics, Eugenics, Embryo Ethics.* Manchester: Manchester University Press.

Strauss, Anselm, and Juliet Corbin. 2000. "Grounded Theory Methodology: An Overview." In *The Handbook of Qualitative Research,* edited by Norman K. Denzin and Yvonna S. Lincoln, 273–85. Thousand Oaks, CA: Sage.

Strørmsvik, N., M. Råheim, N. Øyen, and E. Gjengedal. 2009. "Men in the Women's

World of Hereditary Breast and Ovarian Cancer—A Systematic Review." *Familial Review* 8(3): 221–29.

Strørmsvik, N., M. Råheim, N. Øyen, L. F. Engebretsen, and E. Gjengedal. 2010. "Stigmatization and Male Identity: Norwegian Males' Experience after Identification as BRCA1/2 Mutation Carriers." *Journal of Genetic Medicine* 19(4): 360–70.

Sulik, G. A. 2010. *Pink Ribbon Blues: How Breast Cancer Culture Undermines Women's Health*. New York: Oxford University Press.

Sussner, K. M., L. Jandorf, H. S. Thompson, and H. B. Valdimarsdottir. 2010. "Interest and Beliefs about BRCA Genetic Counseling among At-Risk Latinas in New York City." *Journal of Genetic Counseling* 19(3): 255–68.

Tambor, Ellen S., Barbara K. Rimer, and Tara S. Strigo. 1997. "Genetic Testing for Breast Cancer Susceptibility: Awareness and Interest among Women in the General Population." *American Journal of Medical Genetics* 68: 43–49.

Tercyak, K. P., B. N. Peshkin, R. Streisand, and C. Lerman. 2001. "Psychological Issues among Children of Hereditary Breast Cancer Gene (BRCA1/2) Testing Participants." *Psycho-Oncology* 10: 336–46.Thrush, Sharon A., and Ruth McCaffrey. 2010. "Direct-to-Consumer Genetic Testing: What the Nurse Practitioner Should Know." *The Journal for Nurse Practitioners* 6(4): 269–73.

Trusso, Jennifer A. 2010. "District Court Holds Gene Sequences Not Patentable Subject Matter." Martindale.com. http://www.martindale.com/legal-management/article_Sheppard-Mullin-Richter-Hampton-LLP_979638.htm.

Vadaparampil, S. T., G. P. Quinn, C. Knapp, T. L. Malo, and S. Friedman. 2009. "Factors Associated with Preimplantation Genetic Diagnosis Acceptance among Women Concerned about Hereditary Breast and Ovarian Cancer." *Genetics in Medicine* 11(10): 757–65.

Vadaparampil, S. T., and T. Pal. 2010. "Updating and Refining a Study Brochure for a Cancer Registry-Based Study of BRCA Mutations among Young African American Breast Cancer Patients: Lessons Learned." *Journal of Community Genetics* 1: 63–71.

Van Riper, M. 2005. "Genetic Testing and the Family." *Journal of Midwifery and Women's Health* 50(3): 227–33.

Van Riper, M., and A. Gallo. 2005. "Families, Health, and Genomics." In *The Handbook of Families and Health: Interdisciplinary Perspectives*, edited by D. R. Crane and E. S. Marshall, 195–217. Thousand Oaks, CA: Sage.

Vodermaier, A., M. J. Esplen, and C. Maheu. 2010. "Can Self-Esteem, Mastery and Perceived Stigma Predict Long-Term Adjustment in Women Carrying a BRCA1/2-Mutation? Evidence From a Multi-Center Study." *Familial Cancer* 9(3): 305–11.

Vorhaus, Dan. 2011. "DTC Genetic Testing and the FDA: Is There An End in Sight to the Regulatory Uncertainty?" Genomics Law Report. http://www.genomicslawreport.com/index.php/2011/06/16/dtc-genetic-testing-and-the-fda-is-there-an-end-in-sight-to-the-regulatory-uncertainty/#1.

Werner-Lin, Allison. 2007. "Danger Zones: Risk Perceptions of Young Women from Families with Hereditary Breast and Ovarian Cancer." *Family Process* 46(3): 335–50.

Werner-Lin, Allison. 2008. "Beating the Biological Clock: The Compressed Family Life Cycle of Young Women with BRCA Gene Alterations." *Social Work in Health Care* 47(4): 416–37.

Werner-Lin, Allison, and Daniel S. Gardner. 2009. "Family Illness Narratives of Inherited Cancer Risk: Continuity and Transformation." *Families, Systems, & Health* 27(3): 201–12.

White, Della Brown, Vence L. Bonham, Jean Jenkins, Nancy Stevens, and Colleen M. McBride. 2008. "Too Many Referrals of Low-Risk Women for BRCA1/2 Genetic Services by Family Physicians." *Cancer Epidemiology, Biomarkers and Prevention* 17(11): 2980–86.

Williams, Shawna. 2007. "Myriad Genetics Launches BRCA Testing Ad Campaign in Northeast." *Genetics & Public Policy Center Newsletter 23.* http://www.dnapolicy. org/news.enews.article.nocategory.php?action=detail&newsletter_id=26&article_id=111.

Williams-Jones, Bryn. 2006. "'Be Ready against Cancer, Now': Direct-to-Consumer Advertising for Genetic Testing." *New Genetics and Society* 25(1): 89–104.

Wilson, Brenda J., and Holly Etchegary. 2010. "Family Communication of Genomic Information." In *The Handbook of Genomics and the Family: Psychosocial Context for Children and Adolescents,* edited by Kenneth P. Tercyak, 163–89. New York: Springer.

Yale Cancer Genetic Counseling. 2010. "Myriad Raises Price of BRCA Testing, Again." *Yale Cancer Center Genetic Counseling Program Blog.* http://yalecancergeneticcoun-seling.blogspot.com/2010/04/myriad-raises-price-of-brca-testing.html.

Zikmund-Fisher, Brian J., Angela Fagerlin, and Peter A. Ubel. 2010. "Risky Feelings: Why a 6% Risk of Cancer Does Not Always Feel Like 6%." *Patient Education and Counseling* 81: 87–93.

Zola, Irving. 1975. "In the Name of Health and Illness: On Some Socio-Political Consequences of Medical Influence." *Science and Medicine* 9(2): 83–87.

Zola, Irving. 1977. "Healthism and Disabling Medicalization." In *Disabling Professions,* edited by Ivan Illich, 41–68. London: Marion Boyers.

Index